Jum & Muz

I Forget - A Caregiver's View of Alzheimer's

Jum & Muz

I Forget - A Caregiver's View of Alzheimer's

M.E. Connelly

Jum & Muz: I Forget A Caregiver's View of Alzheimer's
Copyright © 2021 M. E. Connelly

Printed in the United States of America

First Printing 2020

M.E. Connelly
1603 Capitol Ave, Suite 310 A552,
Cheyenne WY 82001

ISBN: 978-1-7379626-4-9 (Paperback)
ISBN: 978-1-7379626-5-6 (Hardcover)
ISBN: 978-1-7379626-3-2 (eBook)

To James (Jum)

We cannot understand many things; fathomless questions that confront and confuse us, but the most baffling is the human mind. I have shown my observations, interpretations, and explanations with additional notes I found helpful with that thought in mind.

I hope this book will remind us what a kind, sweet, considerate, and compassionate person Jim was. Thank you to my family for being the thoughtful, caring people you are. And to Jim's friends, a special thank you. I could not have survived without your help and inspiration. His life ended much too soon.

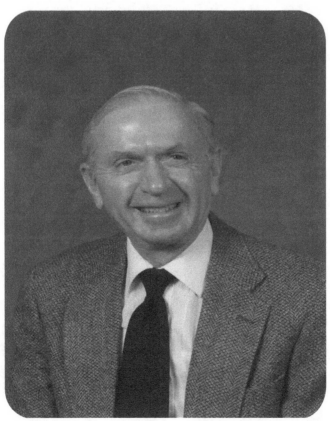

Jum

OLD IRISH BLESSING

May the wings Of the butterfly kiss the sun

And find a shoulder to light upon-

to bring luck, love, and happiness

Today Tomorrow and Beyond.

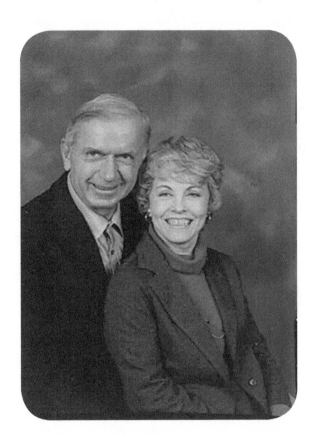

Jum & Muz

TABLE OF CONTENTS

M. E. Connelly

I Forget----A Care Givers View Of Alzheimer's

Alzheimer's has been named the cruel disease, and this is true. It sneaks into the brain and steals the dignity, memory and sense of self of the person affected. It begins with a small, insidious loss of consciousness, maybe misplacing keys. Wondering why did I go into a particular room? What was the reason to enter that room, what did I need, why did I come here? Unease and frustration is an early sign. At first, maybe it's just the thought that this is a (so-called) senior moment. Everybody has those. It's terrifying to feel like your memory is slipping, and you can't think as clearly as you once did. This story portrays my husband, James' gradual descent into the oblivion and unforgiving grip of Alzheimer's. The devastation the disease caused our family, but especially to him, we lived it.

My husband was a thoughtful, brilliant man. He had a great sense of humor and enjoyed a good joke. He loved to tell stories to make people laugh. He had an unbelievable store of limericks, I'm sure, some he made up himself. Jim was a people person in the best sense of the word. His thoughtfulness was apparent, especially with children and dogs. He enjoyed a game of solitaire that he invented because he said the conventional method was boring. He read everything and anything. He could quote poetry or a line from a book to cover any situation. His mental acuity was genuinely outstanding. But over the course of about twenty years, his mind gradually retreated behind a cloud of panic, frustration, uncertainty, and debilitating worry.

1

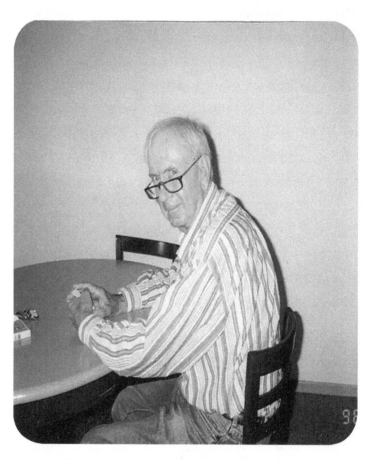

Jum, Playing Solitaire

The most devastating part of dealing with someone enduring Alzheimer's is not knowing what will happen next and when. The gradual personality change flashes back and forth. The bewilderment of the person affected is, I think, the most heart-breaking part of the disease. You feel such sympathy, but there is nothing you can do except try to cope each day. The progression of the disease is insidious, and the sense of isolation and loneliness is sometimes overwhelming. As a caregiver, it is a burden you carry alone.

A friend once asked me how I stayed in a marriage with such a problem. I guess my first thought was a shock that someone could think that way. You do not abandon someone if you care about them. I thought how, each day, there was another reminder of the loss as the disease progressed. Our memories together, our shared memories, are now gone. I read somewhere that Alzheimer's has been called "The Long Goodbye." That is an apt statement of fact.

The isolation can be overwhelming if you let it. You need a support system. I did not realize this at first, and I tried to handle the problems and incidents alone. I did not ask for help. However, several organizations offer assistance and information I did not have. The Alzheimer's Association is an excellent source of information. Their research is gaining insight into the cause, and studies are underway on how the disease might be prevented.

My children were married, living their lives, and I did not tell them early on. If they did not see him often, they probably would not notice the changes. But in the later stage, they were helpful. However, I did not know what was happening for quite a few years. It did not appear essential to tell them, mainly because I did not know myself. I did not investigate options until much later as the disease was further along. I had not been familiar with Alzheimer's. Finally, I studied, searching for information and research, but not until it became evident that something was wrong. The symptoms quite often go unnoticed until the disease has advanced significantly. Some warning signs seem ordinary until you realize they are coming more frequently. They are so unusual that you finally have to notice, they are not typical.

The changes were minuscule at first and were few and far between. Because the episodes were irregular, sometimes months would pass. I didn't always notice a change in behavior or activity. I thought Jim was tired and attributed it to the long hours on a freight train. He was a locomotive engineer on the Great Northern Railroad. He was absentminded occasionally, but that did not appear to be anything for worry. We all have those moments, you see. However, I understood the occasional flashes of anger. But he was not an angry person, so I speculated about what had upset him. How Could I fix it? I was successful some of the time.

I think it's necessary to present some background of Jim and our family to better understand the circumstances of dealing with the effects of Alzheimer's. I was twelve when my parents divorced. My brother, Melvin, the oldest, was married of the seven siblings, and Evelyn, the oldest sister, was also married. While living in Coram, Montana, my Dad was successful in a bid on the Railroad section in Sandpoint, Idaho. Following the divorce, two older sisters Vera Mae and Dorothy, stayed with Dad. The three youngest sisters, Helen and Charlotte, and I went with our mother when she moved back to Montana.

My mother remarried, and because Charlie held various jobs, we moved several times. Charlie bought 160 acres north of Whitefish, Montana. Along with my two youngest sisters, we moved to the Big Mountain on the turnoff road toward the Whitefish Lookout. It was a log cabin, very rudimentary, with one big room and a loft, part of the original homestead.

Without electricity, we used kerosene lanterns for light. A wood-burning cookstove with a warming oven above the cooktop furnished our only heat. We did not have running water, but there was a spring about 50 feet from the house. My stepdad, Charlie, installed a hand pump and a barrel to catch the water; it was not as inconvenient as it sounds. We did have to heat water for dishes or clothes or baths, which were a pain. My mother groused about the three of us not helping enough, but we were kids and needed reminding. We had a washing machine with a ringer to force the water out of the clothes. It had to be wound by hand and did not do a good job. Consequently, the clothes took a long time to dry. Of course, we did not have a drier, but a clothesline served.

Without a car, our only form of transportation was walking or horses and a wagon. Much later, Charlie bought an old truck. The cab was exceedingly high. Consequently, the windshield had a hinge across the center. The radiator had to be drained every night during freezing weather to avoid the block freezing and cracking. It was essential to use a hand crank to start the engine. It seemed to me we had a flat tire every time we needed to go somewhere. And, because tires had a rubber inner tube, the tire had to be removed. The inner tube had to be patched and filled with air again. I guess everyone had a hand pump, just for such a purpose.

Jim was born in Whitefish in 1926 and grew up on the lake side of town. He had three older sisters, Shirley and the twins. Jim loved fishing. During the depression, he sometimes supplied dinner for the family because his father (Jay) was laid off and out of work. With Whitefish beginning to recover from the depression, the men furloughed were now back to work. Jay was hired back as a Locomotive Engineer on the Great Northern Railroad. In 1938 when the Lakeside school burned to the ground, Great Northern officials provided a railroad car as a classroom while a new school was under construction.

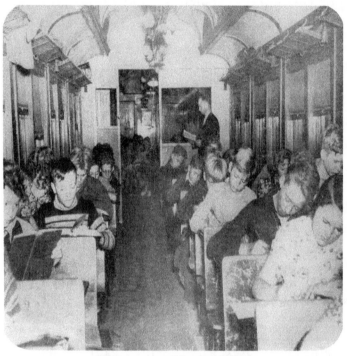

(Classroom on Wheels – 1938)
(Jim – 3rd up on right- blond hair, white shirt)

A group of Lakeside boys had a running feud with the town kids. Jim told me they made slingshots out of old rubber inner tubes and had wars shooting rocks at each other. It's incredible to me that nobody was seriously injured. An older boy lived across the street. Hugh was the unofficial leader of Jim and the boys (Rex, Larry, and Harold), and he looked out for them and kept them out of trouble. Following graduation from High School, Jim immediately joined the Navy. Boot camp training was at Farragut, a base near the small town of Sandpoint, Idaho. How strange, my family lived there during the Japanese attack on Pearl Harbor and our entrance into the war raging in Europe. I was ten years old.

Returning to Whitefish following discharge from the Navy, Jim attended the University at Missoula on the GI Bill. He changed his major several times and struggled to decide what he wanted to do. After we were married, Jim transferred to Billings and began the curriculum to teach. He thought 7th grade was the ideal age to have the most influence on young minds.

Although I didn't know it at the time, I first encountered Jim when my sisters and I walked down a back road. The road down the mountain was an old wagon trail, mostly ruts, and rocks. We went a few times a week to get milk from a dairy farmer a mile or so from our cabin. We took Jinks, our dog, with us because Mom was worried about bears. It was probably a legitimate worry, but we couldn't have cared less and pooh-poohed the idea.

Jim told me many years later about seeing us one day. He said he was returning from a fishing trip, and he saw one of the three of us drinking from the jug with milk dribbling down her chin. That summer was unbearably hot, and my sister, Helen, always gulped some of the milk before we arrived back at the house. Our mother's scolding did not affect her. Helen continued to do it even when I reminded her she was going to get a talking-to. I guess she figured it was worth it because she always pushed to the edge. She hasn't changed in the years since, not just the milk issue but almost everything she did.

In 1946 Charlie traded the cabin on the mountain for a house in Whitefish a half block from the lake. A tremendous change, we now had running water, a bathroom, a telephone, and electricity. Because we were used to adversity; (it was a three-mile walk to school), we did not consider the distance a problem. Even after-school activities required us to walk if we wanted to be involved. However, I didn't have time for anything extra at school. My only school endeavor was a reporter for the school paper. During my Junior and Senior years, I worked an hour every afternoon in the Superintendent's office. My job was to answer the telephone and update the files.

In October of my Sophomore year, the Commercial Class teacher recommended me to the Pacific Power Company Manager. I was hired and began work as a telephone operator. My shift was every day after school from 4 to 8 p.m. and 8 hours on Saturday and Sunday. I walked the three miles to and from the telephone building. My starting wage was 34 cents an hour, and when I quit five and a half years later, I was making a dollar and ten cents an hour.

Looking back, I missed many fun things while attending school, such as football and basketball games and other activities. My schedule allowed only one prom, my Junior year. During the summer months, I worked a 40 hour week until school began in the fall. I graduated from High School in the spring of 1949, and my employment with the power company increased to full-time.

In1946, 1 started my first job. However, I had not applied.

I was a sophomore in high school enrolled in the commercial curriculum. The subjects included typing, shorthand, and bookkeeping, which supposedly would be preparation for a job and a good foundation for employment. My chances of going to college were nil.

The school had a strange system. If you planned on attending the University, you took one set of subjects. If you didn't plan on attending a university, you signed up for a different set of topics. The university prep classes included calculus, geometry, chemistry, and physics, to name a few. Girls were discouraged from taking those classes. Girls could take Home Economics. Boys not planning to attend college could take shop.

I didn't know the school had counselors. And at the time, I didn't realize I was seventh in my class, and you could talk to someone about a curriculum. At the time, I was covering school events for the "Bulldog," the school newspaper. It occurs to me that the school must have had dismal information outreach since I didn't know about these things.

Towards the end of October, the Commercial teacher asked me to come back when classes were over. I went to her room at four o'clock, and she introduced me to a man sitting by her desk. He was the Manager of Pacific Power. He seemed very pleasant, putting me at ease with a few casual comments. Did I enjoy school? Did I participate in sports? Small talk. I had no idea why he was there and why the teacher wanted me to meet him.

"I'm looking for a student to work after school and on Saturday and Sunday. I asked your teacher for a recommendation, and she suggested you might be interested." After a short interview, I was a telephone operator.

The first day was an orientation given by one of the operators. The switchboard was an old PBX, the kind with cords and plugs. When someone wanted to place a call, they would pick up their receiver, and a light would flash on the board at the telephone office. The operator connected one end of the plug, ask for the number and push the other end into the connection for the number called. The majority of the lines were party lines. Some had four, and some had six or eight. On the lines with more than one telephone, the number also had a letter to signify the second telephone. A few private single lines were available for business or government telephones.

For example, if your number was 214, you answered one ring, but you answered two rings if it was 214X. If the number was 214Y, you answered three rings, and so on. Of course, you were only to answer your call. Consequently, some people listened in, and privacy wasn't an issue. It was a small town with only a few hundred phones.

The Manager scheduled an assortment of shifts. Two women with seniority worked day shifts with an overlap from split shifts during the busiest times. I worked after school from four until eight. Weekends and during the summer, I was listed for a split shift. One split was 7-00 to eleven a.m. and 3-7p.m. Another was 11 a.m. to 3 p.m and 7 to 11 p.m. The operators did not like the divided shifts. They broke up the day. You couldn't plan anything because you had to be back at work. We lived three miles from the telephone building, and without transportation, I walked those miles, sometimes several times in one day.

Occasionally I might be lucky and get the 8 to 5 shift, with an hour for lunch or, my favorite, noon to 8 p.m. One woman worked the night shift - 11 p.m. to 7 a.m. and said she liked having the daytime available. But of course, someone had to do her two nights off. The other operator's schedules were for those on a rotating basis.

On a summer evening, I answered a call from the Sheriff. He asked if I would monitor a phone number and let him know the conversation. I agreed, and the next day I mentioned the call to the Supervisor. She said it was illegal. Because I did not know that, I had some apprehension about what would happen. I hadn't listened in on any calls. The Supervisor said she would contact the Sheriff. She also said he should know it was illegal to ask an operator to monitor calls. I didn't hear anything further, so I guessed I wasn't in trouble.

On a Friday, the night operator was sick, and the Manager said he needed me for the midnight shift. I had been at school all day, so I went home and tried to sleep instead of working my regular four to eight. I was only fifteen, concerned whether I could handle it, let alone stay awake.

The first night wasn't a problem, I nodded off about 3 a.m., but I drank lots of coffee and splashed cold water in my face. Saturday night, however, was a disaster. I must have fallen asleep because I heard banging and shouting, and all the lights on the board were flashing. With the night alarm and the fire siren screaming, the noise was deafening. It took a few seconds to get oriented and remember where I was. I was so scared I was shaking when I went to the door. A fireman, who had been pounding the door, looked enormous in his fire gear, His face turned beet red, and he yelled: "I've been trying to get you for about twenty minutes." One of the operator's duties was to turn on the town siren when notified of a fire. He continued to yell. "I drove down here to set off the alarm myself when I couldn't raise you. There's a roaring house fire, and the firemen are trying to call in." Because we had a volunteer fire department, the firemen would call the switchboard to learn the location. Usually, this system worked.

After I calmed down, I fretted and paced and drank coffee for the rest of the night. I worried I might have caused someone to lose their house or, even worse, their life. The fire turned out to be mostly smoke damage, but that experience was so frightening that I never fell asleep again when I worked the midnight shift. After I met my future husband, Jim would call, and we chatted during the night shift. The switchboard was mainly quiet, and those conversations kept me awake.

Interestingly, the second year I worked there, the Power crew joined a Union, and the operators could also belong. An insurance plan included one clause that caught my eye. It stated; pregnancy was not covered because it was a self-incurred disability. Although a few of us might have wanted a clause that included pregnancy and other women's issues, the operators laughed. Insurance has not changed much in that respect.

I worked the midnight shift many nights when I should have been going to school activities. Child labor laws must have applied to my situation, but my parents couldn't have known. The teacher never followed up, and I didn't complain. It didn't occur to me that I could. Nevertheless, it was a learning experience. That first job helped prepare me for my entrance into politics, listening as a basic necessity.

The following year, when we were married, I continued at

the phone company that summer. My husband, Jim, was piling brush for the State Forest Service. However, we spent many hours discussing our future and what we would do. The GI Bill was a perk for his service in the Navy. He served on a Yard Mine Sweeper in the South Pacific. Because he enjoyed children, our decision, Jim would pursue a goal in teaching. Following the transfer from the University at Missoula to Billings, I quit my job. He also worked part-time at the Catholic Hospital as an Orderly. I was not working because we were expecting a baby. I didn't expect to be as homesick as I was, but we had each other. When the GI Bill ran out, we moved back to Whitefish, intending to return to the University when we saved enough to do so. That plan never materialized when Jim was hired as a Fireman and then promoted to Locomotive Engineer on the Great Northern Railroad. With a steady income and three children, it made more sense to stay in Whitefish. Occasionally we discussed whether to return to the first plan.

I joined the local Woman's Club, part of an international service organization, and was elected President and then District President. I was also covering the City Council and school board meetings for the local newspaper. Those experiences eventually led me to politics. I campaigned for and was elected to the Montana House of Representatives. I served five terms, appointed by the Speaker, on the powerful Appropriations and Budget Committee.

Additionally, I was appointed by the Appropriations Chairman to serve as chair of the Long-Range Planning Sub-committee. I served on several boards and Committees, such as the Alcohol and Drug Abuse Prevention Council. Because my district bordered Canada, I was appointed to the Economic Advisory Council, consisting of Montana, Idaho,

Oregon, Washington, Alaska, and Alberta, Canada. That first job certainly helped prepare me for a future in politics. It was a learning experience. It taught me how to deal with people, be responsible, and how often things we do affect others.

Two

One summer afternoon in 1949, a friend who lived next door invited me to a movie. He said a pal of his would meet us with his date. The guys were home for the weekend from the University at Missoula. When introduced, I was surprised when Jim said, "I've already met you." I found this to be a rather strange **statement because I had not seen him before that day. A comment by** Larry changed the subject before Jim could elaborate. It wasn't until much later he told me about seeing us on the mountain road with the milk jug. It was a strange thing to remember, I thought, but interesting, nevertheless.

He was six feet tall and rather skinny. The first thing I noticed about him was the piercing blue of his eyes. They held your gaze so you couldn't look away. Throughout that summer, we went on several double dates. I discovered Jim lived at the end of the block from my house. It seems odd that we had not crossed paths before.

One day in late summer, I was at the post office, and Jim came in as I was leaving. We chatted a few minutes, mostly small talk about the heat and the forest fires and if the weather would ever change. The hot, dry weather had created a tinderbox, and the whole state seemed to be on fire. Smoke and haze drifted in a low cloud, adding to the intensity of the heat.

He invited me for coffee. We sat for several hours, reminiscing about the summer discussions and the various movies we had seen. He called the next day, and we met again for coffee. We spent occasional afternoons at the lake. After a quick swim, we enjoyed lounging in the sun. Whenever we were at the beach, my dog came along, and if we were in the water, Jinks guarded the towels. He started doing this when my sisters went to the lake. We hadn't told him to stay, and he just seemed to know it was his job.

Jim and I went on long walks talking about everything; movies, books, the galaxy, authors we liked or didn't like, but mostly just enjoying each other's company. Working the midnight shift (which sometimes happened) trying to stay awake; always dead silence and boring. I mentioned this to Jim, and he called in one night. After that, those midnight talks helped to pass the time.

After several dates, we thought we should tell his friend of our interest in one another. It was becoming much more than just friends. As we got to know each other, I realized he had a keen intelligence and a warm, appealing manner. He was outgoing and never condescending. We discussed friends, our families, our plans for the future, everything.

One of the incidents Jim told me was about his sister. Home for a weekend from the University, he discovered Shirley and a friend had painted his Model A lavender. After I met Shirley and we became friends, she told me about how sorry they were. Jim was visibly upset with them, and Shirley said it wasn't as funny as they thought it would be. They agreed to repaint the car black. Later Jim sold the car when he needed money. He told me selling it was probably a dumb idea because we could have used a car after we were married.

During our long talks, he elaborated on the crazy things they did as kids. He said all the boys started smoking. When he was eight years old, he had his first cigarette, a habit that continued off and on until he was in his sixties. Smoking added to breathing problems, and I'm convinced cigarettes contributed to the later diagnosis with Emphysema. The diesel smoke from the locomotives contributed, as well. I'm not proud of it, but I nagged him to quit smoking. Eventually, he did, but only after years of stopping and starting again and again. Of course, smoking was an additional health issue we coped with because the Emphysema grew worse as time passed.

The labored breathing probably limited him physically to a certain extent. He had trouble walking any distance after several years. To me, it seems reasonable that a causal relationship exists. Regular physical activity increases oxygen to the brain, which, in turn, supports better cognitive performance. However, it was many years before the Emphysema limited his movement, forcing him to walk slowly. It also caused him to stop often to catch his breath.

Over several years I noticed a lack of interest occasionally in things he enjoyed. Apathy may mean the brain is changing. A lack of interest and energy may signal a drop in brain activity. Episodic memory is the type that typically diminishes – the ability to remember specific events. The Hippocampus is the brain area that usually shrinks in people with Alzheimer's. Studies are underway to find how to help preserve it. Research has also shown brain tangles. A picture of a healthy brain alongside a picture of a brain undergoing Alzheimer's changes shows a drastic difference in composition.

Jim borrowed his parent's car, and we were married later the following year. It was a simple wedding where my parents lived in Sandpoint, Idaho. Helen was my maid of Honor and a family friend, the best man. Mom baked and decorated a lovely cake, and Charlotte, my youngest sister, served. Surprisingly, my step-father seemed visibly moved. I didn't realize he was that emotional. But when thinking about his reaction, I remembered his anguish when two Marines delivered his son's ashes. His son died in the Bataan death march during the war. Not the same, of course, but emotional nevertheless. A few tears amid hugs all around.

Leaving, following our wedding, the car broke down while we were driving toward Spokane, Washington. A fish salesman with a freezer van stopped to offer help. He chauffeured us to our reservation. When told we were just married, he offered a bottle of champagne. I told him I wasn't old enough to drink, and he said flowers would work. A stranger to us, but a nice, thoughtful guy. I don't remember what was wrong with the car, maybe out of gas.

Back at Whitefish, we had to think about our future instead of just dreaming. We considered various ideas trying to decide what we wanted to do. We were drifting, and our options seemed limited, but we were young and in love. The world was our oyster, so to speak. However, our optimism and spirit of discovery could not foretell the coming events that would change everything. Throughout the trials, tribulations, and turmoil, our life together lasted fifty-one years.

Three

The first year of our marriage, we rented a small furnished apartment in downtown Whitefish. I continued to work at the Telephone Company, and Jim spent that summer piling brush for the Forest Service. We were still considering various options. We had discussed our ideas and plans before, but we had to get serious about our future. The pros and cons of staying in Whitefish made that future seem rather bleak.

Following those discussions, going back to the University seemed to be the best option. Having decided Jim should go back to school, I quit my job, moving to Billings. Our only possessions were clothes and a few books, so it was a stress-free move by bus. However, it was scary because we didn't have enough money to last more than a few weeks. Our circumstances could have been dire. But we were looking forward. I wanted to conceal my worries from Jim, but I think he sensed my concerns because he held me and made soothing comments.

Jim transferred from Missoula and enrolled at the University in Billings specializing in teacher training. He reactivated the G I Bill available to Veterans. Jim served during World War II on a yard mine-sweeper in the South Pacific. Our plan, to continue toward a degree in Education he had begun while at Missoula. Because money was in short supply, he worked part-time as an orderly at the Catholic Hospital. I was expecting our baby, so I wasn't looking for work. We thought if we scrimped, we could get by okay, and we did, for the most part. We were both products of the depression, so we were learning how to conserve. But learning how to make

19

money last through the end of the month took some trial and error. Laughter was a saving grace, and we laughed a lot. Better to laugh than complain.

We rented a small one-bedroom house on the back of a lot convenient to the Hospital and University. The owner was a nurse at the Hospital. Shortly before we moved into the rental, the woman told us her neighbor had lost their seven-year-old daughter. Hit by a car and did not survive.

The nurse had two little girls, and they came to visit every few days. They mostly came to see Jim, I think. The three-year-old had trouble pronouncing James, and she began calling him Jum, and the nickname stuck. I started calling him Jum, and later on, our children called him Jum, as well.

We were practically destitute, so, of course, we didn't have a car. On infrequent occasions, we hired a taxi. We were often down to a loaf of bread and ice cream during the last week of the month. I have since questioned whether the university's chronic stress contributed to the later memory loss and confusion. It seems there might be a correlation, but I have no evidence to base it on.

When our son was born, it became more of a struggle. I spent seven days in the Hospital. Since I didn't have anyone to help, the doctor told me that I needed to recuperate after a 23-hour labor. Visitors were not allowed, except husbands or mothers. The nursery had a diarrhea outbreak and was still under quarantine. However, when the doctor discovered Jim worked at the Hospital while attending school, he waived his fee. The Hospital also relinquished charges. Their decisions lifted a terrible burden from us.

Once in a while, I would visit, and the nurses cooed over our son, Jan. They teased Jim about his child bride. I was nineteen but looked twelve. One day a priest passed me in the hallway and stopped to comment about Jan, "he's so beautiful, there's something special about him, you should enter him in a baby contest." I think the priest was joking, but it was a pleasant thought, nonetheless.

We walked to the grocery store every Friday, located eight blocks from our house. We put Jan in the buggy and made it an enjoyable part of our day. We usually took the same route and passed a house with a small terrier. He probably weighed 10 or 12 pounds. If outside, the little dog ran out and barked. He was cute but an irritant. One day the owners were sitting on their front porch when the dog ran toward us. He nipped Jim on the back of his leg. Without thinking, Jim turned, raised his foot, and caught the dog under his belly. Jim lifted the dog into the air and tossed him about 20 feet toward the porch. The people didn't say a word. The dog was not hurt, but he yipped and ran up the steps. Funny, he didn't run toward us after that. He sat and barked from the safety of the porch.

Jim's cousin Virginia (Chris) and her husband Earl were also attending the University. Earl had red hair, but it was actually a light shade of Pink, so, of course, his nickname was Pink. They had a car, so if we were desperate for a ride, they were available. Jim and Chris were very close because she lived with Jim's family throughout high school when Virginia's mother died. Another strange phenomenon. As I mentioned before, they lived at the end of the block from my house. Chris was two years ahead of me, but I hadn't seen her outside of school even though we attended at the same time.

The second year in Billings, we drove to Whitefish for Christmas with Chris and Pink and their baby girl, a few months old. We stopped at a service station for gas and a snack. Returning to the car, Chris remarked, a shoebox has disappeared from the back window ledge. She started to laugh. When we asked why she was laughing so uproariously, she said the box contained dirty baby diapers. "I don't use a diaper bag," and that was convenient; just put the whole stack into the wash. We joined in her laughter, and Earl commented, "Somebody will sure have a shock when they open that box, probably expecting a fancy pair of shoes." Still laughing, we continued on our way.

It was starting to snow when we left Billings. Unrelenting, the snow turned into a blizzard and increased in volume as we turned toward Seeley Lake through the Swan. It was drifting and blowing into ridges on the highway. Earl said he hoped we made it through before it was too deep to navigate. As we got closer to the junction at Bigfork, the snow stopped. The temperature was dropping, and the highway was snow-packed and slippery. The Highway Department had not plowed the main road, so we were concerned about getting stuck in a drift. Earl said, "I hope we make it to Whitefish before it freezes." Just as he said that we slid into the ditch. By trying to steer out of the snowbank, we were forced in deeper with the wheels spinning. Earl tried to rock the car out of the drift with no success.

The guys got out and looked at the snowbank. Deciding there was no way out of this dilemma, we sat a few minutes, contemplating our situation. Jim suggested he go to a nearby house and ask to use their telephone to call a tow truck. We all agreed that it was a good idea. Jim and Earl proceeded to the house while Chris and I waited. A few minutes later, an older woman came out of the house. She had a parka loosely over her head and shoulders, and as she approached the car, she said, "You should come in out of the cold. It's freezing, and the wind is picking up, and you can't sit here with youngsters. Come on now."

We trooped after her as she led the way to the side door. Earl was on the telephone, and the lady told us to hand her our coats and sit down by the fire. We did as she said, settling into chairs facing the fireplace. Earl said it would be a couple of hours before the tow truck would arrive, and we would be stuck in the ditch for a while. The lady's husband came from the kitchen with hot chocolate and cookies. He said, "No problem – you stay as long as necessary. We enjoy the company. And besides, where would you go anyway?" Jim chuckled, and Earl said, "That's true, and thanks for the hospitality. We appreciate it." Indeed, it was four hours before the tow truck arrived to get the car out of the ditch.

We were very late arriving in Whitefish, and Jim's folks were worried, even though we had called to explain. Over the next week and a half, we enjoyed being fussed over and spoiled. The trip back to Billings was uneventful, and we returned to the drudgery of school and work, looking forward to spring break and a change in the weather.

Part of the curriculum for a degree in Education was practice teaching. Jim spent several weeks as a fourth-grade practice teacher. The school was on the opposite side of town from the University. The area, a low-income section of Billings, is primarily immigrants and Hispanics. The kids loved him, and when he concluded his time at the school, the kids planned a going-away party with cupcakes, a piñata, and balloons. It was apparent they had spent a lot of time planning. They had music and songs, and one girl read a poem she had written about Jim and how he had inspired them. I attended the party along with Jan. They fussed over him, cooing and patting his head, and one little girl offered to hold him, "He's so cute," she said.

As the party concluded and we were preparing to leave, some of the kids cried, I cried, the teacher cried, and everybody cried amid hugs all around. Even Jim appeared moved by the love flowing over us. He told them to stay in school, study hard, and mind their teacher. You can do whatever you want to do because the future is wide-open. He told them he hated to leave and how much he would miss them. They all yelled, "Me too, me too, me too."

Jim was still working part-time as an orderly at the Hospital; we struggled with a baby, schoolwork, and a limited amount of money. The Veterans program funding ended, and without that income, we had to make a decision. We thought Jim should finish the school year, but we looked at the cost, and there was no way we could swing it. Much soul-searching convinced us we were short of options. We moved back to Whitefish. Because we were living in a furnished rental, we didn't have much to move, clothes, baby stuff, and books. A final cleaning and we were ready. Without a car, we scrounged a ride with Jim's cousin Chris and Pink. Chris said they were planning a visit to Whitefish, so we were not an imposition.

Four

It seemed strange. We were back where we started. Without jobs, no money, and no place to live. We stayed with Jim's folks a month until we found a house. After a few months, Jim was hired as a Fireman on the Great Northern Railroad. Later, management promoted him to Locomotive Engineer. We always intended to go back to the University and continue the original plan to teach. But, with the security of a job Jim enjoyed, the program didn't materialize with a regular paycheck. We settled in Whitefish permanently. Even the best of intentions sometimes go by the wayside. From time to time, we discussed the idea of going back and felt sad we hadn't made more of an effort.

The schedule of the railroad was crazy and a continual upheaval. Jim was on call after eight hours and could be on a trip for sixteen to eighteen hours. After a long trip the off time was only eight hours, no matter how long on duty. In January, the second winter, Jim was sent to Essex to keep the tracks open on the snow machine. The way had to be cleared. As a result, over the winter, the snow piled in huge drifts. The heavy trains climbing the steep grade over Marias Pass and the Continental Divide needed a helper engine. Depending on the number of trains, the Helper crew might work four, eight, or ten hours. The temperature dipped below zero and stayed for several weeks. The snow piles froze and packed into solid ice, and fresh snow added another hazard on top of the ice. The discharge from the diesel smoke coated the snow with streaks of black soot.

The weather stayed below zero, and In the house we were

renting, the water froze. I was added to a waiting list to get thawed out. Everybody in town had frozen pipes, and the waiting list was lengthy. Jim had not been able to come home for over a month, so I was left to handle all the trouble caused by the piercing cold. I had shoveled snow high up against the house, but still, the water froze. It was incredible. On a short visit home, he was sympathetic but couldn't do anything to help in the small amount of time available.

The extreme cold dissipated, and the temperature climbed to 20 degrees. The wives of the crew at Essex decided to go for a visit, kids and all. We boarded the passenger train for the short trip from Whitefish. The Isaac Walton Hotel, owned by the railroad, provided for the crews stationed at Essex. We spent four days at the hotel where the men stayed while they battled the snow. We saw the guys only a few hours at a time before they had to be back to work, sometimes for sixteen to twenty-hour shifts. The long hours took a toll, I'm sure, and they must have been exhausted. I know I was. Jim did such a fantastic job on the snow machine; management assigned him to Essex the next year and the next. The guys nicknamed him 'The Snow King.'

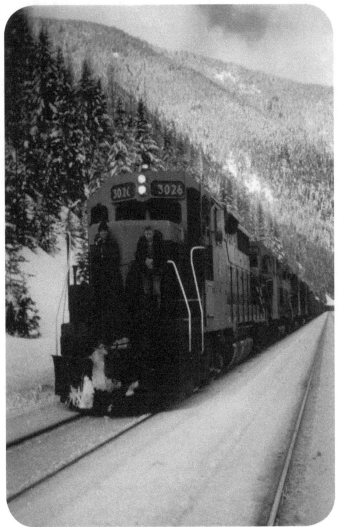

GN locomotive – Marias Pass – Jim

My brother lived only a few miles from the Continental Divide but worked out of Essex. Melvin operated the Jordan Spreader and the front-end loader. Mel was such an expert with the loader that he could pick up a raw egg and place it without breaking it. Mel was legendary along the district. The rotary plow threw snow into high piles beside the tracks, and the berms froze solid. Mel had to dig out along the banks where the rotary threw snow. Even following the spring thaw, the ridges seldom melted for months. Finally, the crew at Essex returned to Whitefish and the regular schedules of the trains.

Tired of renting, in 1957, we bought a small house on the road leading to the Big Mountain ski area and resort. When I say small, I mean tiny, 900 square feet, one bedroom, and an unfinished loft. We had three kids, Jan was seven, Becki was four, and Pat was two months old. So, until we added a kitchen and half-bath, we were crowded. Finishing the loft gave us more room to expand. Life was simple, with our three kids and Rusty, a Cocker Spaniel.

Moving to the tiny house, we were five miles from Whitefish. After she crashed a few times, Becki learned to ride a bicycle. The kids rode bikes if they had something scheduled. Jan rode to baseball practice every Saturday, and later Pat joined a team. We attended all the games, including Jim's childhood friend, Hugh. Becki brought her friend Ruth. Becki started calling me Muz for some unknown reason and it wasn't long before Ruth did as well. Then the boys decided if Beck could address me as Muz instead of Mom, they could too. Consequently, Muz became a nickname I still have to this day.

A friend from the railroad brought an English Setter to our house. He said his brother in Illinois raised registered purebreds, and Art thought they wanted one of the puppies. Art said they couldn't do anything with her and would we take her. Being soft-hearted, we did. She was named Queenie, a beautiful dog but never fit in with Rusty, the Cocker Spaniel, or our family. She was a basket case, scared of her own shadow or a loud noise, frightened of everything. She cowered in a crouch if inside. She was afraid to walk across the kitchen. Her nails clicked on the linoleum, so Jan carried her back and forth.

Somebody dropped off a dog by the side of the road, near our house. We would have adopted her. She appeared hungry, and the kids brought her into the house to offer food and water. However, when we took her to the vet for a checkup, he said she was in bad shape. He couldn't save her. We only kept her a week, not even time to give her a name. I wonder why some people are so irresponsible. She was a beautiful dog.

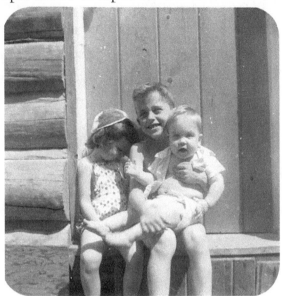

Log House
Becki, Jan, Pat

The young couple who built the house used logs they cut and notched themselves. They used a block and tackle to lift the logs into place for the walls. I was amazed and impressed when they described their efforts, and the result was pretty extraordinary. An interesting aside – I was staining the logs and had about a half gallon leftover and decided I might as well use it up. We used an open shed on the back of our four aces for storing wood for the heater. I painted the posts. During tax season, the assessor came by, noticed the shed, made a note, and added it. Apparently, the county had not included the woodshed in the tax form. So much for my idea to be thrifty and use up the last of the stain. All it did was increase the property tax.

Jim found a kitten one day and brought her home when he came from work early. We were all delighted, and he said to the kids. I have a surprise, but you have to look for it. Becki looked at him for a few seconds and then reached into his pocket. She jerked her hand back and then gingerly put her hand in again and pulled out a tiny kitten. Jum said the freight train was stopped on double track, waiting for the passenger cars to pass. He saw the grass moving and went down to look. He found the kitten, but there was no sign of a mother. He searched but did not find her.

The kitten, mainly dark gray, had diagonal black stripes on her back and legs. We fed her with an eye-dropper until she was big enough to eat on her own. Jan named her Pooella. He said a friend of his told him that meant "little girl" in Russian. We didn't know if this was true, but it was a good story. Pooella grew up to produce four babies twice a year. It became a running joke to find someone to give a kitten. It got to the point that if I called a friend or neighbor before I could say more than "hello," I heard, "No, I don't want a kitten," and hung up.

Pooella did have one saving grace that people appreciated. She had seven toes on all four feet. At least one of her many babies in each litter had an extra toe on one or sometimes two feet. She loved to play with string. She used her paw like a fist. She could throw a marble against the wall, catch it, and throw it again. Unbelievable what she could do with those extra toes. A boy delivering a weekly newspaper stopped one day and asked if he could show his friend 'the weird cat.' The friend was adequately impressed, and Pooella became notorious in the neighborhood.

A friend of ours had a hobby of creating homemade wines. Art experimented with new additions. We were visiting one evening, and he said he had a new wine he wanted us to try. The primary ingredient was Rye, and he thought it had promise. We agreed to take a bottle, let it sit for a month or so, and try it. Then he wanted us to let him know what we thought of it. I laid it flat because he said to keep the cork wet. Jm was called to work for a freight train to Troy and left around eleven. I went to bed and was awakened out of a sound sleep by Pooella screaming, Meow, Meow, Meow, Meow, Meow. She was charging up and down the stairs and continued the cater-walling at a high pitch. At the top of the stairs, she was carrying on, still running up and down. I smelled a strange odor. It was sharp and piercing and hurt my nostrils. I was at a loss as to what was causing such a nauseating smell. I went downstairs. The odor was more apparent when I entered the kitchen, and I followed the stench into the pantry. The bottle of wine had exploded and blown the cork. The wine was everywhere, on the counter, the ceiling, the cabinets, and the floor. I was so angry that if Art had been there, I think I might have strangled him. It took hours to clean the mess. The bottle was empty. Later, when I explained the explosion, Art was apologetic and said he probably would not try that wine again. I agreed and told him I did not want to test his products in the future. He said that was a good idea. But it was rather funny after I calmed down enough to think about it.

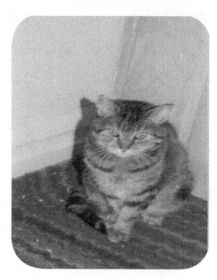

Pooella

Eventually, Pat (he was ten at the time) called the veterinarian and set an appointment. We were all grateful. No more kittens to try to find homes, as he stated emphatically, "I'm tired of losing friends." Pooella lived to be 25, and we were all saddened when she died following a stroke. The vet told us Pooella was her oldest senior citizen. It seemed as though Pooella was with us forever, which in a strange way was true; she had been part of our family for so long.

When Pooella died, the kids had already married and moved to their own homes, and I called to tell them. I was concerned. Everyone was in a funk. I worried that Jim might take it hardest because he was becoming more easily agitated. At the time, I didn't realize it was probably the memory loss and the increasing frustration. I wrapped Pooella in a towel, and we buried her in the backyard. I said a prayer to myself, and I cried when he began to shovel dirt to cover her tiny body. Jim seemed unusually quiet. Pooella was such a character and so special to us. It took me a while to settle back to a semblance of normalcy.

I missed her curling up in my lap. I stroked her as she purred softly before going to sleep as she had for so many years. Pooella was strange in many ways. I was babysitting my nephews' baby while he went for a job interview. I had Logan on my lap (he was sound asleep) when Pooella decided she wanted her space back. She tried to push between the baby and me, tried to push him off my lap. She followed me when I put the baby into his basket and waited for me to sit down. Then she climbed up on my lap as if to say; this is my spot. No babies allowed.

Jim's empathy and affinity for understanding relationships carried over to the railroad. The young guys his age went to him for advice. They asked about the job or girls or any crisis in their lives. Quite often, one of the guys would stop for a chat and stay for an hour or two. One particular incident still troubles me after all the years that have passed. One night around three in the morning, I awoke to a knock at the door. One of Jim's friends from the railroad stood there. He looked distraught when I told him Jim wasn't home - he was on a trip to Troy. I asked if he wanted to come in and have a cup of coffee. He stood in the doorway a minute or so. I mentioned again, come in for coffee, but he mumbled that maybe he would be in touch and left. A few days later, I learned he had killed himself. I often think of that early visit. Could I have done something? Should I have been insistent that he come in for coffee? What if Jim had been home? Because Jim sensed what it took to soothe a troubled co-worker, could he have helped and perhaps saved the man from his ultimate suicide? That thought still haunts me. The stress of the odd hours on the railroad affected the wife of one of the Firemen. She had two small children, and she put them outside, locked the screendoor, and shot herself.

Why she did not ask for help, nobody knew.

I mentioned the men at work, but Jim was equally at ease with children and dogs. They gravitated to him like a moth to a flame. I marveled at his patience. My nephew loved to fish, and Jim took him along sometimes on a fishing trip with our kids. Jim helped with Cub Scouts and coached Little League. He taught Becki (our daughter) to fly fish, and she was as skilled as the boys and loved it as much as they did.

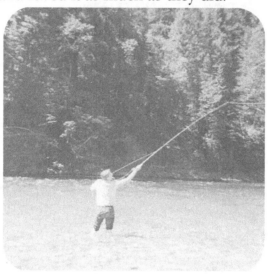

Jum – fishing the North Fork

We were only about five miles from the ski resort, so we bought a season pass as a family. Lots of fun, and the kids took to it immediately. For Becki's ninth birthday, we gave her a complete set of "Heads," the premier ski at that time. Her eyes went big, and she was ecstatic. We invested in new skis for everybody the following year. With a season pass, you could ski every day, and if the weather was lousy, quit early and hope another day would be better.

One winter, the snow melted earlier than usual. The traffic up the mountain created a gigantic crater in the road in front of our house. The first car was stuck, and those following couldn't get through. They lined up five or six deep. The farmer down the road offered to pull them through, and the various drivers agreed. However, while this was happening, our cat, one of Pooella's babies, the big yellow tom, walked back and forth, over the hood and the roof, leaving paw prints. Some of the drivers thought it was hilarious, and others complained. It took me a while to coax him off a car. I apologized but thought it was funny.

We skied together as a family until the boys left for college. Becki and I skied one season every day. She was attending Flathead Community College so we could take a half-day every day. Pat and I skied one day on his rare day at home from Bozeman. We stopped to rest, and Pat yelled at me to get out of there. Kids jump from the jeep trail above. Before I could move, a boy came off a jump (which was prohibited) and knocked me end over tea-kettle. I tumbled and slid 300 to 400 yards down the hill. Skis, poles, my hat, goggles, everything flew. The kid was panic-stricken; he kept asking me, lady, are you all right? I didn't know. Pat said the kid must have had tremendous reflexes because he turned his skis in mid-air and hit me on the back sideways. Pat said if the kid hadn't rotated them, he would have knocked my head off. A disconcerting thought.

Pat and I quit for the day. We stopped at the Beer Stube, and the kid was at a table. As we ordered, the boy lifted his mug. With both hands shaking, he tried to raise it but spilled some of the beer. I wondered if he was in any condition to drive down the mountain. As a result of the collision, I experienced a torn cartilage in my knee. I gave up skiing after a couple of years (too painful).

In late March of one year, when the snow was melting, the sun was shining, and it was a beautiful spring day. My friend Shirley and I had a glorious time but quit early. We decided to go to the Beer Stube before starting for home. The place was empty except for the two of us and a man at the bar. We ordered a couple of mugs and sat down at a table.

He came over and asked if he could join us. He said he was a reporter for the Chicago Tribune doing a story on the mountain. He asked if we were locals and when I said yes, he asked if we would answer a few questions about the ski runs and Whitefish and the Flathead. We agreed. He sat down with us and started by asking about the Big Mountain, the type of snow, the crowds, and fees.

Shirley responded, and I listened, marveling at her long, drawn-out description as she explained. It was a crappy area. The snow is either too wet or too icy and consistently awful. She elaborated on how terrible the conditions were, and the wind blew constantly. The charge for a day was too high. It eliminated too many people. The food was rotten because nobody seemed to care. If you rented equipment, the chances it would be old and probably out of date were more likely than not. She didn't have a good thing to say about the ski run or the lifts or how the mountain was groomed.

She elaborated on Whitefish about the high rates at the motels. The road to the Mountain was treacherous, and the switchbacks were too sharp. Traffic up the hill was always slow and dangerous. The reporter asked numerous follow-up questions, took many notes, finished his beer, and thanked us before leaving.

Shirley broke into hysterical laughter, "I guess I told him.

Maybe people will read the article he writes and will never come here. I want to keep this ski slope uncrowded and economical."

We giggled at the idea that he probably believed us. Later, in May, I was at breakfast, following the service, to welcome a new priest to the Episcopal Church. He made the rounds of various tables, chatting with everyone. I asked him where he was from, and he said Chicago. He mentioned he had done some research before considering moving to Whitefish. He said he saw an article in The Chicago Tribune and was interested. But, he told me he was a little apprehensive after reading it because of the negative connotations about the area. He said the article quoted two women he had met on the Big Mountain. They were vehement about the lousy resort and the Flathead generally. I explained to him at length the encounter my friend and I had with the reporter that Shirley wanted to keep the area to ourselves without advertising it. We had a good laugh about the story, and my family became good friends with the new priest.

Another time Pat was knocked down when the chair swung around too fast and knocked him off the platform. He was six at the time and was very indignant. He told the operator to learn how to run the thing or find another job. The guy said he would do that.

Shirley and I took the chair most of the time. She swung her skis as we went up the hill. While we were chit-chatting, I gestured with one of my poles to make a point. The pole caught the cable and stopped the chair. We swung back and forth fifteen or twenty minutes before service was restored. As we skied off at the top platform we heard someone say, "It was some dumb woman, swinging her pole that stopped the lift."

We pretended not to hear and skied off down the mountain. Shirley kidded me about that episode now and then.

Four veterans built the Big Mountain ski area, and one of the original veterans skied well into his nineties. He taught at the high school and served as Principal and later as Superintendent. He was a tremendous influence on the young people in Whitefish. Several others were involved as well, both with the school and the Big Mountain. Skiing the Big Mountain was a great family experience we enjoyed.

With our hectic school and activities, sports, and music schedules, I insisted our evening meal be a family event, if at all possible. I wanted to know what was happening at school. If they were having problems, anything that might be out of the ordinary. With Jim at work for days, sometimes weeks at a time, this was very important for continuity and connection. Mornings were too chaotic for any serious thoughts or comments. The school bus came early, and it was always a mad rush. Becki had kindergarten three days a week. She rode the school bus in the morning, and I picked her up at noon.

My niece once told me, "I liked coming to your house for dinner when Uncle Jim was there because the jokes and discussions were so much fun. Everyone had a chance to say what they thought without interruption or ridicule." Whether talking about school or the current political issues, those conversations were far-ranging. Sometimes rather loud and quite often tongue in cheek. We solved the problems of the world while chatting around the dinner table. A joke could spark a burst of hilarity. Laughter dominated our conversations at times but always veered back to meaningful observations. Those family dinners continued for years, and the kids have repeated that tradition with their families.

The political discussions were always the most involved. I was active in local politics, belonging to the Democratic Central Committee and working on campaigns. I served as a volunteer for years, at headquarters, making phone calls, stuffing envelopes, and whatever candidates needed.

Five

A few years later, in 1964, we built a house on Glenwood Road and moved again. Moving from four acres to a lot in a neighborhood took some getting used to. We were much closer to town, and the lake was only a few hundred yards below. The contractor agreed to defray a portion of the costs; we could do the sheetrock and painting. Jan was thirteen, and he offered to take over the cooking while we spent long hours at the construction site. He became a fantastic cook. He searched cookbooks for new recipes and ideas. During this time, following one of Jan's spectacular meals, Jim commented, "All the kids should learn to cook." He chuckled when he said, "otherwise, they could look in a mirror and watch themselves starve to death." Of course, this caused everybody to laugh, but all three learned to cook.

The construction seemed to take forever. Finally, with the house finished, we built a fire in the fireplace. We toasted with snacks and hot cider. Pooella kept going back to the old house for several weeks but finally adapted. The two dogs accepted the move. Anywhere we were, they wanted to be. Even Queenie was adjusting.

Queenie began bringing things home; a shoe or a glove, or a dish. She carried halved milk cartons from next door. The neighbor had planted seeds, and they were dumped, with a trail of dirt to our front door. The boys took turns taking things around, asking people if something or other belonged to them. Queenie developed a tumor and died the second year at the new house. We felt sad. But she had never become part of the family, the way Rusty, the cocker, or Pooella had.

Queenie didn't overcome her fears; nothing we did helped her. We thought she must have a psychological problem, maybe because she was purebred and inherited a trait of some kind.

Moving from the tiny house to a four-bedroom took adjusting – we rattled around for a few months. It was a pleasant house. But, even though closer to town, not very convenient to church or the projects and interests the kids developed.

Jan worked every summer throughout high school. He was employed two summers in Alaska for Alaska Packers. Later on, weekends were spent washing dishes at a restaurant. Another summer, he did handyman work at a Resort. The resort owner stopped me at the grocery store one day and told me Jan was a pretty spectacular kid. The man said he didn't have to express what was needed; everything just got done; he's reliable. Jan also clerked at a clothing store. An item of interest at the store. Jan grabbed a shoplifter in the act, and the owner was so grateful and impressed, he gave Jan a raise.

Pat spent one summer laying ballast on the railroad and another summer helping a friend change irrigation pipe for a farmer down the road. Pat worked with a local doctor for eight weeks before beginning pre-med. That September, Pat transferred from the Flathead Community College to Bozeman. A club member of mine mentioned that she was scheduled for surgery but was frightened of the outcome. She said Pat sat with her, explained the procedure, and he would stay with her and be there when she woke up. A truly remarkable young man, your Pat is. I am eternally thankful he was there when I needed somebody.

In 1971 I took a shortcut on a back road; I discovered a farm for sale when returning from a meeting. We checked it out and immediately liked the house, the outbuildings, and the area. Consequently, we sold the residence on Glenwood and moved again. Three kids, two dogs, and Pooella. (Did I forget to mention we now had a Chesapeake Bay Retriever) a friend of ours raised. Becki wanted a dog of her own, so she picked a litter's runt and named her Ginger.

The first year at the farm, Pat planted a vegetable garden, and it was beautiful. However, when he dug up the potatoes at the end of summer, he found stumps of roots or a potato half-eaten. The gophers had a field day with their free lunch. The following year he gave up on the garden. Ginger loved searching for gophers. You could see her rear and tail halfway out of a hole as she dug. She never caught anything, but we didn't discourage her.

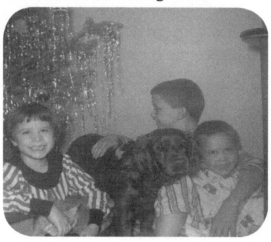

Becki, Jan, Pat

Throughout the growing-up years, all three of our children participated in activities and did odd jobs at various times. Our daughter worked with a horse trainer, took lessons in dressage, entered exhibitions, and won blue ribbons. In exchange for the training, she spent afternoons and Saturdays mucking out stalls and grooming the horses.

Pat later joined a rifle club. Jan and Pat were active in Cub Scouts, Boy Scouts, baseball, and band. All three took piano lessons and had featured solos in a recital. For a few years, Jan and Becki took dance classes, including tap. The instructor had a presentation program every year. The parents and grandparents, and friends attended, and it was standing room only.

The boys served as acolytes in the Episcopal Church, and Becki sang in the choir. Jan was one of the acolytes for the ordination of a new Bishop for Montana. Because the Episcopal Church in Whitefish was too small for the expected crowd, the church hierarchy performed the ceremony in the Catholic Church in Columbia Falls.

Becki was the narrator for the Christmas program for three years, beginning when only six years old. Pat wondered how she had the courage. He said he would be too scared, but it didn't bother her. She had total confidence in herself, and that confidence never wavered.

It seemed strange that Pat questioned her courage. He had no qualms about anything, such as a piano presentation, participating in a shooting meet, or performing a horn solo with the school band. One year the ensemble (of which Pat was a member) was invited to Washington DC to join in a concert with the United States Army Band. I still have the recording provided to each of the students.

Jan was equally confident in Boy Scouts or a solo in the district sectionals for the school band. He was a National Merit Scholar, the top 1% of students nationwide. All three were honor students, probably because they loved school and enjoyed extra-curricular activities. Reading was a priority at our house. Life was frequently unorganized but fun and satisfying.

Jan was married and attending the University in Oregon, so he did not live on the farm. We enjoyed the visits home with their two children, Lara and Jeff, and their dog Champ. Champ was intimidated by Pooella, and as he came in the door, he charged upstairs to avoid her. He was terrified, and we had to protect him from the cat. He was a Pomeranian, so she was almost as big as he was.

Not long after moving to the farm, our Cocker Spaniel Rusty, age seventeen, began wandering. He was going blind and consequently couldn't find his way back. We found him after the initial search. But if we didn't watch him every minute, he wandered away again. One day I couldn't find him. We searched for hours, and I placed an ad on the radio about a lost dog, and a lady brought him back. The next time he got away, we could not find him. I'm convinced he wanted to go off somewhere to die. It's difficult to lose a beloved pet, especially in such a sad way. When Ginger died at age sixteen, we found another Chessie at the pound. She was ten months old, and we named her Bo. She was a one-person dog (Jum's) and very aggressive. A tremendous but unpredictable watchdog. We received the newspaper by a carrier, and he came once a month to collect. He was so afraid of Bo that he stayed in his car and blew the horn until somebody came out. I agreed with him about Bo. However, the UPS guy wasn't afraid, and when I asked him why, he said, "I always carry a carton of cottage cheese for the unruly dogs. It works great." True, Bo could hear the truck coming a mile away, and she would sit by the driveway, waiting.

In 1980, visiting with Evelyn, Babe, and Dorothy, we discussed a family reunion. We decided Memorial Day would be the best time, and I suggested the farm. We had lots of room. I contacted Helen, and Abby offered to roast a half-beef on a spit over the outdoor fire pit. Becki and I sent invitations, and over 200 people responded. Some of the relatives we had never met, so it was fun to get acquainted. The BBQ was fantastic, but the weather was lousy. It was an overcast day and only 65 degrees. It had been 80 the day before. My nephew rigged up a tent with a tarp and set up the guys' kerosene heaters used for ice fishing. It was a perfect day, even though the weather didn't cooperate.

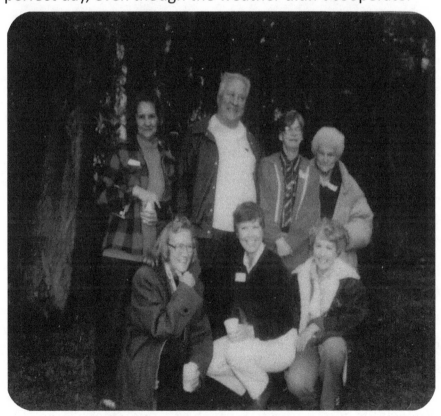

Family Reunion 1980—Charlotte took the picture
Evelyn, Melvin, Dorothy, Mom
Babe, Helen, Mary Ellen

The 115 acres had initially been part of a homestead. The house, built in 1914, was two-story with a full basement. The property also had several outbuildings. The chicken coop was an eyesore, the garage needed a roof, but the granary was excellent. The barn was enormous and had a recent roof replacement but required paint. It had a huge loft for hay storage where pigeons hung out by the dozens. We laid out a schedule of how to proceed to update. We fell in love with the farm. The rhythm changed in different ways, Becki and the horses; Pat and the rifle meets, and, of course, music and school. It became a small hobby farm, as the CPA called it on our tax return. We later planned to sell parcels as a resource toward retirement. We raised barley and alfalfa, then leased the acreage to a farmer on a percentage basis.I say this merely as background for the beginning of the condition, later diagnosed to be Alzheimer's.

The work on the farmhouse proceeded as planned. The first year, Pat and a friend shoveled the old wooden shingles off and installed cedar shakes, replacing the leaky roof. Bill was laying the shakes, and Pat followed with the staple gun. We heard a scream, a crash, and then a brief silence. Pat had stapled Bill's boot to the roof. When Bill realized it had gone between his toes, they started to laugh. Pat had to pry the boot loose with a crowbar. We joined the laughter when they told us what happened. In the process, they removed the lightning rods. We discussed their necessity, which turned out to be short-sighted when a thunderstorm flashed lightning through the house, doing extensive damage. It melted the telephone connections into a mass, burned off one side of the TV connections, burned the wiring on the washer on one side. It had to be programmed halfway through a cycle. It burned the wiring in the garage, but not the wiring to the pump in the well. It blew the top off a cottonwood tree, throwing the top across the yard, and it stuck into the ground like a spear. We replaced the lightning rods again.

We remodeled the obsolete kitchen, painted, added tile, and new carpet in the living room.. The walls in the living and dining rooms consisted of wallpaper that looked like canvas. With lighter spots where pictures had hung, we decided to paint it. A guy with knowledge of this type of paper suggested using varathane to cover the spaces before painting. We did as he told us, but the wallpaper shrunk and separated, and then we had a hideous wall, with strips of open area. We had to sandblast the walls to remove the paper and replaster before we could paint.

The first winter, when the wind blew, snow drifted in around the wall sockets. You could sit on the sofa and watch it blowing across the room. Insulation became a priority, and later, replacing the siding. The wood siding was full of holes from woodpeckers searching for dinner; the knotholes formed a pattern where the birds had destroyed them. After replacing the siding, I happened to be outside when a bird flew up to the house and hit the new siding. The bird slid down the wall but must have been shocked. He could no longer search for insects.

Before adding new siding, we insulated, hoping to curtail the snowdrifts across the rooms. After investigating, the best option seemed to be blown-in foam. The idea was to cut several holes in the outside walls and feed the liquid foam into the walls. Supposedly it would spread around and harden as it set up. The installer suggested I go to an upstairs bedroom and yell if the wall began to bulge. I hollered, but the man didn't hear me, so I had to run down and warn him to stop. Then he had to repair the bulge in the inside wall. Eventually, under the siding, during replacement, they installed plasterboard. The new siding got rid of the holes made by the birds and the insulation guy.

Pat was taking pre-med at Bozeman. The first semester, if he planned a weekend home, he called to ensure the heat vent in his room was open. The furnace was an oil burner, probably ninety years old. Old and crotchety and took forever. If the wind blew, it was drafty and impossible to heat the house. We invested in heavy socks and wooly sweaters. We did not replace the furnace but installed a new burner. We added a fireplace with a blower, and the ambiance heated the living room and dining area. It did not help the upstairs, however.

One afternoon Jim was called to deadhead from Whitefish to Spokane, WA. They were to return a freight train to Whitefish because a crew wasn't available on the other end. En route to Spokane, the train derailed near Colburn, Idaho. Several cars tipped over and jack-knifed into the bank. The deadhead crew was tossed around and thrown to the top of an upside-down car. Jim was hit in the head and knocked unconscious for several minutes. He also had a severe back injury. The crew was off work only a few days. It boggles the mind when I think about it.

Later, we talked about the dangers of working on the railroad. Jim said his biggest worry wasn't a derailment or a broken rail, but a logging truck getting stranded and hung up on a crossing, unable to get out of the way of the oncoming train. A collision of that sort happened much too often, causing death and injury, not only to the crew but to innocent passengers or bystanders if it happened while passing through a town. People are much too careless about railroad crossings – ignoring warnings and signs. People could prevent the resulting injuries and tragedies with a bit of common sense and attention. Most people don't think about the amount of time it takes or how far a distance for a train of over 100 cars to stop. Even though only going 20 or 30 miles per hour, it could take a mile or more if the boxcars are loaded with produce or other products. Flatbeds or empty boxcars also need an incredible distance to slow or come to a stop.

Although I had seen signs earlier, I now think that crash with the resulting concussion was probably the beginning of the brain damage that resulted in the onset of Alzheimer's. It almost certainly contributed. The proof is continuing to build in that direction. Studies of football head injuries are a case in point.

After the kids graduated, Jan was married and attending medical school in Oregon. Becki was taking classes at the Community College and working for a law firm. Eventually, all three were married, moved away, and had started families. The memory episodes were not occurring very often. **B**ut Jim seemed more bothered by pressure at work and happenings on the farm. It didn't seem meaningful, but I noticed occasional spurts of anger or anxiety, frustration, and bewilderment. Sometimes an irrational statement flared up for no apparent reason, and he would subside into silence. He would sometimes ask a question, and although I answered, he might ask the same question a few minutes later. These occasions happened only rarely, but I began to make a mental note of how often.

Jim's niece invited us to the wedding of their daughter. At the time, they were living in Hayden Lake, Idaho, and we drove over. The wedding was lovely, with baskets of white flowers and bouquets along the church pews. The reception for the family was at their house. We were reluctant to leave with good food and stimulating conversation, but Jim's schedule required him to be at work the next day. It was around eleven o'clock when we finally left their house.

We stopped for gas at a truck stop near Hayden Lake. I was driving, and as I pulled out of the station, I noticed a semi moving out at the same time. I turned toward the highway ahead of him. I didn't want the truck in front of us on the narrow two-lane leading to Sandpoint and Highway 200 toward home.

Approximately ten miles down the highway, a black pickup passed. I didn't think anything about it until he slowed down, slower and slower. The semi was coming up close behind. The truck was within a few feet of our car with his lights on bright and shining full force. As the pickup in front slowed, another pickup drove up beside us. We were boxed in, and I had to stop when the vehicle in front stopped. I had nowhere to go.

The driver of the pickup in front got out and walked toward our car. He was huge, with a beard, plaid shirt, and jeans. I rolled down my window and asked, "What's the problem?" He said, "when you pulled out of the gas station in front of the semi, your husband gave the truck driver the finger." I said that might be true, we were coming from a wedding, and he might have had too much to drink. The guy walked around to the passenger side and told Jim, "You should be more careful about who you're giving the finger." Jim didn't seem to comprehend what the man was saying. I hurried to intervene, telling the man we would absolutely be more careful in the future. He snarled, "You better, or you'll be sorry."

He strode belligerently back to his pickup and drove off. The truck beside us moved off and followed him. I let the semi pass. We waited. The scariest thing about what happened was the reality that we were in the middle of nowhere. Nobody knew where we were. After I stopped shaking, I thought that the guys probably had CD Radios in their trucks and could communicate anywhere along the road. We would have no recourse with anything they wanted to do. This frightening confrontation happened a long time before cell phones. There was nothing we could have done.

After we waited for a half-hour, I drove toward Sandpoint and the junction of Highway 200 toward Kalispell, Montana. All the while watching for a pickup parked by the side of the road. I checked my rearview mirror every few seconds. I was increasingly worried that the incident might not be over. My thoughts kept going back to reality. No one knew where we were. No one would be aware of whether we arrived home until the following morning. If Jim didn't show up for his shift on the railroad, because he was always on time, someone would notice. I thought about contacting the Highway Patrol, but I only had the color of the first pickup, no license plate numbers at all. Telling family members, they were aghast, as was I.

It had been a long time since a significant memory episode, so I was utterly unprepared. We were on our way for a visit with Becki and her family in Seattle. I paid attention to our location if Jim was the driver since he was lost a few times. Occasionally he couldn't remember the road where we lived. I thought that might be a memory lapse like everybody has now and then.

As we turned onto a street that was not familiar, I asked,"
where are you going? I think we turned the wrong way. " Jim
became flustered and agitated. "I don't know where we are.
Why are we here? Where are we?" I told him we should pull
over and get reoriented as to where we were. I reminded him
we were going to Becki's. However, it took him several minutes
to realize what I told him. He became his old self and no longer
questioned our reason for the trip.

Looking at a map, I located the direction to go, and we
reached the right street and their house. Later that day, because
this was a time he questioned himself, he asked over and over
what was happening. "Why can't I remember where we are?
Why are we here?" He was agitated, and I tried to soothe his
fears, and he soon forgot he had asked. The rest of the visit
was uneventful. Jim was alert, and we enjoyed the time with
them. But, returning home, there was no reason to think about
the Seattle episode.

Another time, while on vacation in Las Vegas, leaving the
airport, he couldn't remember which direction to turn for the
downtown casino area. He was upset and agitated. At this
point, I decided I would do the driving if we had to go any
distance. He agreed without argument. Coming from a man
who had always had a fantastic sense of direction, I think the
frustration and anxiety were beginning to overwhelm him. It
bothered me to see him so upset.

A year passed without an occurrence. Because of the
incidents' randomness, you gain a false sense of tranquility,
thinking nothing unusual happened. I found myself doing this
a lot because it was easy to rationalize. At that time, I'm not
entirely sure if I accepted the totality of what was happening.

Jim asked where we were going; why are we driving a strange car? Where are we? His panic became apparent, and I suggested we pull over, and I would explain. We sat for a short time, and I told him we were going to a casino for a few days, and we could see some shows, and he could play poker for a few hours. He relaxed and soon was no longer anxious and frustrated. We had a wonderful time. Only one peculiar incident caused a minor problem for a few minutes. Jim was playing Keno and using the same six numbers. He said they were his lucky numbers. After eight times without a win, he decided to change numbers. To our total amazement, the original numbers came up. He would have won a thousand dollars. When the initial shock wore off, we had a good laugh about the fickleness of Lady Luck.

I played the five-cent slot machine for a few hours. I kept winning small amounts, and I had my pockets full of nickles. My purse was stuffed, and Jim had his pockets heavy with nickles. We did not have time to turn them in, so I decided to try my luck while waiting to leave at the airport. I ended up losing almost all the nickles. The airport slots were a colossal rip-off.

A year later, while visiting Becki in Seattle, she was scheduled to attend a business conference in late summer. So Jim took a few days off from the railroad, and we offered to babysit. While she was at the meetings, we painted her bedroom and other chores to pass the time. Without thinking it through, it had been so long since a memory lapse; I asked Jim and our grandson, Mike, age five, to go to the corner store. It was only a few blocks away. I needed several items for dinner. They were inseparable during our visits, and Mike knew the way to and from the store. An hour passed, and they hadn't returned, and I was starting to worry. I didn't know the name of the store. I had no idea where to call in a strange town. It was unbelievable that I hadn't asked Mike for the name of the market. I was starting to get an ache in the pit of my stomach. I had random thoughts of what might have happened. Should I call 911? I wasn't sure what to do. I wavered between fear of contacting someone or not calling. Consequently, I did nothing.

It was now several hours since they left. I was picking up the phone to call the authorities when Becki came home. As I explained the situation, Jim and Mike came in the door. Mike said they had been driving up and down the freeway. Grampa was crying and didn't know how to get home. Mike said he talked his Grampa into leaving the freeway. Mike pointed out a place to pull over, and they stopped at a convenience store, but he had no idea where they were. Mike explained to the clerk that his Grampa was upset, and they were lost. He told the clerk he knew his address but not the phone number. He told the clerk the street and said he didn't know where they were or how to find his house.

A customer waiting nearby overheard the conversation. He said he didn't want to butt in, but he knew the area and offered to lead them home. They could follow him, and they wouldn't get lost. Mike told us he repeated to the clerk that he couldn't remember the phone number. He told them he hadn't been able to get his Grampa to stop because he was too upset to listen. The clerk said it was okay, and they would take care of getting them home. Jim calmed down after a few minutes. Mike explained to his Grampa that they would follow the man who said he would drive slow enough; they wouldn't get separated.

When they arrived at Becki's house, the man came in with them. He wanted to inform us why he was there and what happened. He said he thought the little boy had shown such maturity and caring that he needed to tell us. We thanked him profusely, but we were so relieved to have them home that we forgot to get the man's name. I regret that. I thought I should have sent him a letter to follow up, but it was too late by then.

Everything seemed to be back to normal. Life was pleasant but hectic. The memory incidents were few, and I had almost forgotten about them. However, as the days passed, I noticed the lapses and ensuing frustration were coming more often. I was getting more worried because I couldn't help him.

The first of several episodes forced me to contemplate the totality of the problems and how I would deal with them. It compelled me to rethink how to handle what had been happening and was emotionally very upsetting. Trying to overlook the situation was not helpful and added to the stress and nervous tension. I was becoming a wreck. I felt I was losing control because there was nothing I could do to change the situation. I knew it would become worse as time went by. I felt isolated. I was at a loss on how to cope. It was scary as well as unsettling. I called the Alzheimers hotline but hung up before anyone answered. I have no idea why, but I do remember thinking, 'I can't do this.'

A few weeks and another episode occurred. Jan had an automobile at the farm. He was in Oregon attending Medical school, and we agreed to sell it for him. A friend of ours expressed an interest in buying the vehicle. Jim said he would drive it into Kalispell and meet Dave at the courthouse. With apprehension and against my better judgment, I let him go without argument. An hour or so later, Dave called and told me he had seen Jim driving back and forth, but he didn't stop at the courthouse. He seemed to be driving aimlessly. Dave said he would try and catch him, but when Jim finally came home, he said he couldn't find Dave, and he couldn't find the courthouse, "Somebody moved it."

Jim said he was confused and lost and wasn't sure he could make it home. He thought chance had directed him because nothing seemed familiar. He was very disturbed and emotional. I tried to pacify him by changing the subject, telling him what we were having for dinner. I mentioned a few things he liked to do, such as fishing. The lawn needed to be mowed and watered. Anything I could think of that might distract him and help him relax. Nothing seemed to be helping, but I kept talking. Finally, I reassured him enough for him to detail what had happened and what he was feeling. He tried to explain his feelings, but his words were disjointed and didn't make sense. His anxiety took hours to dispel, and he asked me several times how to remember stuff. Why can't I remember stuff? That was a question I struggled to answer.

I was becoming more and more worried. The memory incidents were happening more often and taking longer to dissipate. One day he told me someone was trying to steal his cassette tapes, and he wanted me to call the Sheriff. He thought someone was in charge of our house and the farm. The delusional episodes were only occasionally apparent, and I could convince him that no one was stealing from him. No one was taking over the farm. He said a man wanted us to leave and move off the farm, and Jum was convinced and believed what the imaginary man had said. I could, at times, change his focus if I reminded him of a chore. A few minutes and he forgot the scare he had.

Months passed before there was another major incident. One of the most discouraging things about dealing with Alzheimer's is not knowing when something will happen or what to do when it does. -It's imperative to learn how to cope with the unexpected and unavoidable without falling apart. Probably the most difficult of many difficult things, is not knowing what to expect from a caregiver's perspective. It's easy to push those thoughts aside momentarily, but when they come roaring back, they force you to think. Those feelings are always at the back of your mind. They refuse to go away even though you might bury them temporarily. There's a constant tiny glimmer of fear lurking, ready to jump out at you when you least expect it.

One night Jim came in about midnight and flipped on the light and startled me awake. He left for a trip to Cut Bank only a few hours earlier, so he shouldn't have been home already. Jim borrowed a car to drive back to Whitefish because something had happened at the farm. He didn't know what had happened, but he thought something had. I explained that nothing was wrong, and nothing had happened. It took some convincing, but he drove back to Cut Bank. Jim was scheduled for a return trip and had to be available. I'm not sure he had any sleep since it was a four-hour trip from Cut Bank and another four hours back. He had no memory of the incident and did not remember it the next day.

We hadn't been married very long, so I don't recall exactly how this discussion came about. But, on one occasion, Jim's Dad Jay told us of something that happened to him. Jay had been a locomotive engineer on the GN for over 40 years. He was working on the transfer between Columbia Falls and Kalispell. It was a short run to service business interests along the route. He told us they were going about 10 miles an hour, and a car stalled on the tracks at Columbia Falls. He applied the brakes, whistled the crossing, and rang the warning bell, but the car didn't move. The engine hit the car and shoved it along the rails until Jay could finally bring the train to a stop, a long way down the track.

Jay said he jumped out and lifted an older woman from the passenger seat, and she wet herself and burst into tears. Her husband came around the car, and both were in shock and traumatized. Someone had called, and an ambulance arrived and took them to the hospital, although it appeared they weren't hurt physically. Jay said, after being pushed along the rails by the engine, the car was totaled. He was upset and troubled himself, thinking he could have killed them.

When Jay told us this, at the time, Jim became very curious and asked, "Dad, how can you stop thinking about it?" Forty years later, Jim remembered this story and asked me how Jay could handle the situation so well. He speculated how the accident wasn't more of an issue to Jay. He appeared to be very bothered by thinking about it, and I'm not sure I explained it in a helpful way. Another symptom of Alzheimer's is the flashbacks in great detail to a memory that happened decades ago. However, on the other hand, not remembering something that happened that day or maybe an hour before or sometimes five minutes earlier.

As I mentioned before, he might ask a question and I would answer. But he would ask the same question ten minutes later. If I answered, he might ask the same question again, the same day or a week later. Or, he would tell me something and a few minutes later repeat the question or statement. Jim would not remember he had just told me those exact details a short time earlier. We always agreed with whatever he said. It was much more comfortable, and it helped to keep him calm. By doing this, we kept the flashes of anger at bay, which flared up if someone disagreed with what he had just said. Sometimes the rage made sense, but other times was utterly irrational. Now and then, he would sink into silence for hours. Not moving and not showing a reaction of any sort, no eye movement, no movement at all. I worried that he was not okay. But after a few hours, he sometimes responded to a question.

Seven

After the years away from Whitefish and moving back, I reconnected with my three older sisters. They lived in Fortine, Montana, on Evelyn and her husband, Bob's four acres. Babe and Mom had a house trailer, and Dorothy had her trailer. They split the everyday expenses, such as water and electricity. Jim and I often spent an afternoon visiting. They were pleasant people to talk with, and we occasionally reminisced about our growing-up years. I mentioned one time, I wished I had known them sooner because we spent so many years apart after our parent's divorce.

However, every fourth of July, Mom organized a get-together with family and friends. She had been doing this for over 40 years, and we had a campfire and good food. The guys played guitar, and we always had a sing-along. Sometimes someone would tell a ghost story and cause a minor panic with the little kids. Mom continued to plan the reunions even in later years as her age limited her activity. Although times had changed, they continued; she planned the picnic the last year of her 96 years. However, that summer, there was no picnic. Mom suffered a stroke in December, the year before and was bedridden.

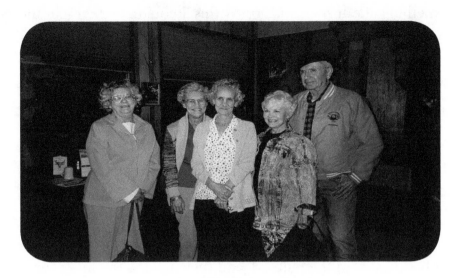

Dorothy, Babe, Evelyn, Mary Ellen, Jum

After we returned to Whitefish from the university, I joined the Woman's Club. The local club had been in existence since the late 1800s. The club was a member of an International Service Club dedicated to building libraries and similar projects. The Whitefish Woman's Club had started the local library. Judy, a friend, was a member, and at her suggestion, I joined in August. She was elected President at the September meeting.

In November, Judy said her husband accepted a position at a Washington University. He taught piano, but shrapnel injuries from the war caused him such pain in his hands that he had to make a change. When she resigned, Judy said she was sorry to leave the club and recommended they appoint me as President. I was petrified, and I think I was in shock. I was so frightened that I couldn't muster the courage to say no.

In the first year of meetings, I was so terrified that I wrote everything down, every possibility of what might come up. I wrote a series of statements to myself. Quotes: If this happens, do this. If so and so says this, answer like this. If someone says something about such and so, say this. I couldn't remember the names of my officers when I had to introduce them. I barely survived the pressure, and I was grateful when the year ended. But it was the best thing that ever happened to me. It laid the groundwork for my future in politics.

I served as President and District President of the local club and Treasurer of the State Organization. During my term as President, I initiated community participation. The club built a warming hut for an ice skating pond provided by the city. Our friend, Hugh, agreed to take charge of the project. He recruited his buddies from the railroad, and they had it done in a couple of months. In a news article from the national organization, my project received extensive praise. Our Whitefish club won a small stipend as a result.

With three children in school, I was interested in the actions of the school board. I attended meetings occasionally. The members on the panel were in the process of deciding on a curriculum that appeared to be unorthodox. Difficult to explain, the discussions gave the impression of being a group think. The Chairman, in particular, was obnoxious and overbearing. He was more interested in power rather than concern for the education of the kids.

Another woman was also concerned. We discussed the upcoming election, and both planned a run against him. She won. Following the election, to our relief, the board abandoned the change in curriculum. Jim commented to me, "I'm proud of you. You guys succeeded; you got rid of him."

In fourth grade, a favorite teacher awakened my interest in politics with a straw vote concerning FDR's re-election. The discussion that followed was in-depth and thought-provoking to me. Consequently, in 1958 I attended a local Democratic Party meeting. I convinced Jim to join with me, and we became involved in local and state politics. I worked for candidates doing the grunt work of helping elect responsible people. We attended the Governor's Ball and other events and dinners. In 1960 I participated in the effort to elect John F. Kennedy. Local Democrats organized, planning fund-raisers and "get out the vote." He won the election, and we were enthusiastic about the new young president and his beautiful family.

I heard the news that morning of the assassination of President Kennedy. Serving as President of the Woman's Club, I called members to cancel the afternoon meeting. To my consternation, a few of the Republican members were upset with me because I canceled. To me, it seemed a sign of respect for the office. It's hard to believe people can be shallow and unfeeling; how could they not be affected by a tragedy so horrible. Jim said it was okay for me to be upset with the women. He was consoling me, but that reversed in later years.

In early May of 1968, I had a telephone call from Washington, DC, a staff member of the advance team for Robert Kennedy. Would I be interested in arranging a meeting to introduce the candidate? I agreed, and he said he would get back to me with the particulars. On the night of June 6th, I watched the gathering in the hotel as the Senator told the supporters, "it was on to Chicago and let's win there." I turned off the television and went to bed. At eleven, Jim came in from a run on the railroad and asked if I had heard of the Senator's death. Jim held me to console me. He knew I was looking forward to the Kennedy visit.

I mentally questioned - is our country coming apart? What are we becoming? What direction would he have taken the country? Would the government be in such disarray if he had lived? The loss of such a unique person is a loss we all share. I grieved for what might have been.

The local Democrats were bewildered as to how to proceed. We needed to reconnoiter. I needed time to overcome my sense of loss. I was uninterested in active political involvement until the early seventies. I wondered if it was worth the effort and sacrifice. I could not shake off the feeling.

However, in a few years, I was still interested and began paying attention to government mechanics. Since fourth grade, in that respect, I could not help myself. Investigating the State Legislature's function and operation, I was concerned, but, maybe fascinated is a better word.

In 1976 I was an appraiser for a law firm. A member attorney was campaigning for the House of Representatives. The staff helped the campaign, door-knocking and stuffing mailers. Following his election, it became necessary to reduce the staff in the firm. I applied for a position as a committee secretary at the State Legislature at his suggestion.

Because of my legal background, I was hired immediately. My appointment was to the Highways and Transportation Committee. As secretary, 1 took shorthand notes of the various committee hearings and transcribed them for the Chairman to review and sign. The minutes became part of the public record and could become evidence, and they had to be accurate and detailed. The rules required that both sides be presented equally. A major committee sometimes had fewer bills depending on the number introduced.

The Speaker of the House and the President of the Senate assigned the bills to the various committees. Each committee individually scheduled the hearings. The action taken by the committee determined several things. A bill could be passed or tabled, or killed. However, a convoluted measure could be sent to a conference committee for revision and also allowed other action. If bills were not acted on in time for transmittal, they would die in committee. A complicated system of checks and balances.

Mid-February, a complex bill was introduced and sent to Highways and Transportation. The legislation required additional inspections and extended oversight of the railroads. Numerous hearings held heated exchanges of opinions and information. The meetings were standing room only, with executives, labor union members, and interested citizens. Sometimes overwhelmed by the arguments, tempers flared.

I took a copy of the bill home over the weekend. I asked Jim to read it and tell me what he thought. He would be concerned because he was a locomotive engineer on the railroad, affecting his job. He asked several questions, and I explained the pros and cons and the arguments presented. He became intensely interested. He thought, reread the bill, then commented, explaining his reasoning, "This is punitive. 1 don't think it would do much good. All it will do is slow up the operation of the train. The inspectors are doing a good job right now. We just need a few more of them to relieve the pressure. This other stuff is superfluous."

If amended, would it be improved, I asked? Several copies had been given to the committee. Jim said the amendments might improve the bill, but it will not do what is intended. I thanked him for his ideas. I was not surprised by his ability to look at both sides of a question.

Returning to the session, I didn't think any more about that particular measure. The Chairman called an executive session for Wednesday evening to dispose of the stack of bills needing action before transmittal. J was there early to set up the room. Several bills were amended and passed. Several were rejected, or tabled, or passed without amendment.

Next, the railroad legislation was brought forward for consideration. A series of amendments offered passed. After a lengthy discussion, the Chairman asked if anyone had any further comments before the vote. I looked around silent, prepared to record the result.

A member from my county asked to be recognized. "Mr. Chairman, I think we should ask the secretary what she thinks. Her husband is an engineer on the railroad, and she probably knows more about it than any of us."

I was startled to hear that and even more surprised when the Chairman agreed, turned to me, and asked, "What do you think about this bill?" I might have stammered my answer. I told them my husband thought it was too punitive. I explained his thinking and pointed out how he surmised the law could affect the operation of the railroad. He agreed with some of the provisions, but they did not do what the law intended. The amendments created confusion. I made a few other comments which I don't remember before subsiding into embarrassed silence The Chairman called for the vote--which was unanimous "Do Not Pass." The bill was killed without further discussion.

It was amazing to me that one person could have that

much influence. I guess knowledge is sometimes the key to determining an outcome. Following the meeting, one railroad official thanked me for understanding the bill's complexities and speaking out against it.

I enjoyed the legislature, returning for two sessions of the House of Representatives.

After serving three sessions as a secretary, I committed myself to run for office. I knew I could do as well or better than the current officeholders.

I had a large group of volunteers, and my brother cooked spaghetti. After wrestling with the pros and cons for several months, I decided to run for State Representative in 1980. The current occupant of the position was not responsive to the people of the district. He didn't return telephone calls or answer letters. I heard complaints from all sides as I laid out my campaign strategy.

Representing approximately 8,500 people, the district covered two mountains and sprawled over a 100-mile radius which included Glacier National Park, Hungry Horse Reservoir , and Big Mountain Ski Resort. Because of the round-about way to get to the Ski resort, the campaign required separate planning for that area. The most populous town was Columbia Falls and included several smaller towns through the canyon.

1 formed a committee of volunteers, led by a republican who was disaffected with the actions of my opponent. "If you can use me, I'll do anything," she said. We laid out a series of advertisements dealing with my opponent's voting record. He had voted against various groups, such as seniors, educators, children, union members, and environmentalists.

A young woman I met during a business lunch came up to me and offered to work full-time as a volunteer. She wrote news releases, contacted people door to door to ask if they would place a sign in their yard. She was a constant source of information and research. We worked out a system. If I didn't remember a name, she would stick her hand out and say, "Hello, I'm Karen." The person would respond by giving a name. It worked like a charm. The district included the Veterans Home, the Plum Creek Lumber Company, and the Anaconda Aluminum Company. The area was a diverse mix. of construction, logging, and low-income. The upper end of the district was at least 60 percent Vietnam veterans. The area was a haven for veterans because no one interfered with them. A friend of mine was a bartender at The Deerlick (a local saloon) and she talked with them from time to time. The veterans were interested in my campaign and volunteered. Meetings at the Deerlick, and we laid out areas where they could help. One particular vet offered to go door to door. Nobody knew his last name. He was called "Walking Steve" because he walked everywhere. He always wore fatigues with a holster on his hip.

He said, "I can talk to anyone, anytime. Let me know where you want me. He said he sometimes had flashbacks to Vietnam, and they were pretty graphic. At such times his face was white and visibly strained..

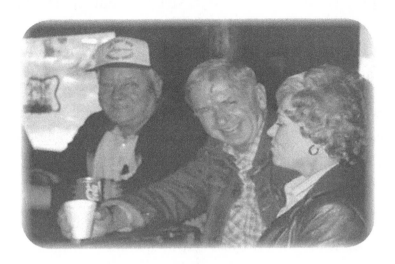

Spaghetti fundraiser, Melvin, Jim, Mary Ellen

The first fundraiser was a Chili feed at the Deerlick. A vet named Dave (a huge man with a full black beard) volunteered the cooking. He was notorious, having fought a grizzly bear with an umbrella. He said he didn't have any kind of weapon. The bear took off. Dave recruited some of his friends to help. My treasurer set up a table by the front door, and a local band offered to play as a donation.

During the fund-raiser, two young women came in, on their way from southern California, back to New England. They said they were interested why all the cars, what was going on? Dave told them he was electing me to the State Legislature. He proceeded to introduce them all around.

They took pictures and said they hadn't dreamed of getting involved with Montana politics. Their friends would probably not believe them, that's why they had to take pictures. They ate chili, drank some beer, and., after a couple of hours, they said they had to go but gave a big donation. The chili cook-off was a spectacular success.

Our second fundraiser was a spaghetti dinner in Columbia Falls. My brother volunteered to cook. My husband's sister, Shirley, donated wine. She owned an Italian restaurant in Spokane.

She said as a bottle of wine was emptied, she put it in her trunk. We were planning to use the bottles as candle holders along with checkered tablecloths. She said she was at the grocery store.

And a boy helped her with the bags. When she opened the trunk, the wine bottles rolled around, clattering against each other. She told us she suspected the box boy thought she was a closet drunk.

Her hilarious rendition of the story started the party off great. The band provided music again, and we raised money. My campaign was off to a rousing start. My nephew volunteered as campaign chairman. He owned a radio station and would plan the advertising.

Plans were laid out on my kitchen table with the core group of volunteers. We developed a brochure and set the schedule for door-to-door visits. Using maps, we divided the area into sections. I went with each group on different days so that I could ask questions myself. I think I had more cookies and cups of tea than any other candidate.

In addition to the weekend door to door, I spent every evening from seven to nine. One evening it started to rain, first a drizzle, then a downpour. But I decided to finish the street. I knocked at the last house, and when a man answered, I told him who I was and what I was doing.

He laughed and grabbed my hands, pulling me into the

house. A lady sat at a table across the room.

"I know who you are," he said, pointing to the woman. "My wife is a republican, but she isn't registered, so that doesn't matter." He handed me a cup of coffee and offered a towel to dry my face.

My hat was dripping, and water was running down my back. "I'm a republican too," he went on," but I'm going to vote for you. I figure that any politician that doesn't know enough to come in out of the rain deserves my vote." He chuckled all the while. We spent a pleasant half-hour, and he told me my republican opponent was useless and didn't care how his policies might hurt. He continued, "You'll be the first Democrat I've ever voted for, and in sixty years, I've never missed an election."

The local newspaper and radio, and TV stations were all convinced my opponent would win by a landslide. A local columnist said I was naive and didn't stand a chance. All the polls showed him winning. My volunteers kept plugging away, working hard, going door to door, answering questions, and passing out flyers. My husband and a couple of volunteers put up signs.

My friend from the Deerlick was poll-watching at one of the Canyon precincts and she told me a bunch of the veterans came in and stomped up to the table, said they were there to vote for Mary Ellen. They all voted and stomped out again, slamming the door as they left. One woman commented "Jeez, that was scary. That doesn't happen every day." Everybody giggled.

The night of the election everyone gathered at my house.

The polls closed at eight. The ballots were counted at the election department at the county seat. Returns started coming in around ten. I carried most of the precincts, but the final count showed him ahead by six votes.

Everyone was discouraged. We sat around for an hour or so,.What had we done wrong or more over what had we not done.

Montana law requires an automatic recount when the vote is within a certain percentage. The recount was carried out at the courthouse. When the recount was complete I had picked up one vote. The result was final, I had lost by five votes.

An interesting outcome, an ironic note, my friend from the Deerlick had four brothers who had gone hunting, with their wives, on the day of the election. When she asked them if they had voted absentee her oldest brother said they hadn't, "Mary Ellen will win, so we don't have to worry." That election proves every vote counts. If they had voted that day I would have won.

I lost the election by five votes, so I was determined to run again. Two years later, I was elected with 68% of the vote and served five terms in the Montana House of Representatives. The Speaker appointed me to the powerful Appropriations and budget committee. In my third term, the Committee Chairman appointed me chair of the Long-Range-Planning sub-committee. The Governor and the Legislature created the Western regional Economic Council. The charge coordinated and promoted cooperation between Montana, Idaho, Oregon, Washington, Alaska, and Alberta. Canada. The Speaker chose me as the Montana delegate because my district bordered on

Canada.

A forest fire, threatening to engulf the area near my brother's home, was spreading rapidly. Melvin was worried about getting his visiting grandchildren out. It was a mile from their house when he planned to evacuate. He had a heart attack, collapsed, and died. The husband of Mel's daughter, Jewel, received a phone call about seven that evening and heard the news about Melvin. He and Jewel decided to go to Essex. When they arrived at the highway, it was closed except for emergency vehicles. The smoke was so thick they couldn't get through anyway. The following day Mary and the grandkids arrived at Jewel's. However, they now had to plan a funeral.

I think the combined worry about the fire and rescuing the grandchildren contributed. Oddly enough, the flames did not reach their house. I had a fundraiser scheduled for that night. I could not cancel because I had no way to know how many might attend. It was an open house. We spent the evening, subdued, trading stories about Mel, with numerous hugs.

We were not close when I was a child. Melvin was much older. But with his help on the campaign, I got to know him and felt a growing affection for him. I was serving in the Legislature at the time of my brother's death. However, this leads to another topic that is necessary to the story of the dreaded Alzheimer's.

Jim's mother, Winnifred, was a character. She absolutely had to clean, mop, and dust every day. We planned a dinner out while we stayed with Winnie and Jay for the month after returning from Billings. When I told her the name of the babysitter, a woman we had known for years, Winnie said, "I can't have her see my house like this; I have to vacuum and mop." I could not see anything that needed doing, but she insisted, so we spent the afternoon cleaning a clean house.

Winnie bowled for years on a weekly team sponsored by the Rebekah lodge. She was left-handed and a power bowler. She had a perfect score many times, and the team received an award from the league. They attended the state tournaments countless times, but I cannot remember if they won or in what order they finished.

Winnie served as treasurer for the City of Whitefish for several years. When I said I was proud of her, she wouldn't acknowledge it as an outstanding achievement. I disagreed and told her so, but she insisted it was not worth mentioning.

During the many years I knew her, Winnie had two health episodes. The summer after we returned from Billings, she suffered an auto-immune attack. Losing weight and became delusional at times, the doctor finally discovered a reaction to a headache pill prescribed for her daughter, Colleen. The doctor sent cultures to the Mayo Clinic to determine the cause and how to treat it. The Mayo clinic recommended he try cortisone with a 50-50 chance it would work. The doctor tried it, and she responded. It took her several months to recover and regain strength. Jay and I mopped and disinfected every day for months. Since she had no immune system, any exposure to anything might kill her. Jay was exhausted, and Jim convinced him to hire a woman to come in and care for Winnie, which took some of the pressure off Jay.

The other matter happened in her 60's. She wouldn't go to the doctor even though she was in pain. She complained of stomach problems for months. She never complained, so this was unusual. Because she wouldn't go to the doctor independently, Jim told her he was taking her. If she refused, he would carry her to the doctor. He didn't have to do that. She did agree to go. She had surgery to remove her kidney. A kidney stone completely engulfed the organ and killed it. She was stubborn, as you may have guessed.

Jim's mother sold her house and was living in a retirement home following the death of Jay. Winnifred had been serving as the night monitor since moving there. Her duties consisted of checking exterior doors, locked with all residents accounted for, that none were absent. If out for the evening, they were supposed to sign back in but sometimes forgot to do so. She served as the monitor for several years.

When she began having significant difficulties, we were concerned. She was giving things away but convinced someone took them. Because she insisted one of the other residents was in her apartment, she was adamant someone had a key. After questioning, we believed her. We talked with the manager, and she said there was no credence to any of the accusations. The manager said Winnie didn't seem interested in acting as the monitor and said she was considering asking someone else to take it over. Consequently, we weren't sure what to believe. We called Jim's sister Shirley in Spokane to ask her opinion.

Shirley and Jim discussed moving their Mother to Spokane. Shirley found a place, and Jim loaded a U-haul for the move. The two of them unloaded and unpacked and arranged her furniture. Winnie began having problems almost immediately, similar to what happened before. It was barely a year when Shirley called and said it wasn't working, and Winnie wanted to return to Whitefish. She was not making friends and was incredibly lonely. So, Jim moved her back and into a Senior

Retirement home. Everything seemed okay for a brief couple of months.

We soon realized she was having delusions again. She told us about strange things happening to her. Someone had a key and was stealing all her stuff. The manager called and told me Winnie tried to pay her rent every few days, even though already paid for the month. The bank called to explain she was having trouble with her finances and someone should help. We decided something had to be done, even though on most days, she was entirely rational.

I called Shirley, and the three of us consulted about a solution to handle the situation. As a result, we bought a house trailer and set it up on the farm. I could be available to look out for her and hopefully intervene if necessary. She would be close by but still have the independence she needed. I took over her finances to get everything straightened out. The bank issues became a chore in itself. Some days, Winnie convinced herself I had taken her money. She demanded her checkbook back. Almost every day, I had to show her where it was in a drawer by her bed. However, she didn't sleep in her bed; she began sleeping on the sofa. When I asked why she said it's because I need my cane for protection, someone might breaks in to steal my stuff. I can give them a good whack, and they'll hightail it out of here.

But I digress. Dealing with the county bureaucracy became an unbelievable nightmare. One county official told me we had to drill another well to accommodate the new residence. In my opinion, this was absurd, and I told her so, but she was insistent. The farm had a well that produced 110 gallons a minute. I tried to convince her there was no way we had to drill another well. But, I could not persuade her. The conversation became heated, and she hollered, and I hollered. It wasn't until I threatened to go higher up that she capitulated and said she would issue the permit. But she disappeared, and I did not see her again that day. Eventually, I received the permit.

On another occasion, I stood by the counter in the county office for several minutes. The employees were sitting, and one guy had his feet up on a desk. They were drinking coffee and making small talk. Being ignored, I finally had had enough, and I raised my voice to ask, " Is someone working? I need information." They looked startled as if I had interrupted something important. The man who came to the counter was wearing a dirty t-shirt, dirty sneakers, and jeans with a gaping hole in the knee

That afternoon I called the county commissioners. I told them it's a disgrace the way the employees dress. I emphasized that if they didn't do something about a proper dress code for the county offices, I was going to raise holy hell. I mentioned it was my opinion that a government office should respect the public, and the people in the office should show that respect. It was interesting. The next time I went to the county office, there was a prominent notice about changes in the way people were to dress and strictly enforced. It was also interesting to see clean jeans, shirts tucked in, instead of grimy t-shirts, shoes, and boots instead of sneakers. I guess the squeaky wheel does get the grease, although maybe the fact that I was a State Representative had some effect.

I still had to fight with Winnie's retirement home about her scheduled move and the county about unnecessary and imaginary problems and issues they perceived had to be resolved. The cooperation was non-existent.

However, to get back to the house trailer. Things had to be done before Winnie could leave the retirement home. I contacted the county to apply for information and necessary permits. I spent days arguing with county officials about permits and inspections. Following the construction, review, and approval of the septic system, I went to the county office to set a time when I would be available for an electrical inspection. The inspector arrived at the farm but didn't get out of his truck.

I asked what's the problem and he said he couldn't approve the electrical as long as THAT DOG is here, pointing at Bo. I told him I could put her in the house. But he was adamant; he couldn't do the inspection and wouldn't get out of the truck. I asked him, "Are you threatening me?" He replied, "Oh, No, No, No." In response, I said, "if you are threatening me, I will call the Supervisors, the newspaper, the television and radio, and anybody else I can think of." He immediately jumped out of the truck and completed the inspection. I finally received an appointment date for the other reviews, done a week later. I got the permits, and all the assessments finished in a little less than a month. Several people told me they had waited months for approval of projects or construction permits. As a State Representative, it's fantastic how things work out with a little bit of influence.

Eight

Winnifred settled in, although she was irrational at times. She used a walker because of unsteady balance. But, always looking down, we had to watch that Winnie didn't bump into things. I couldn't convince her to look up as she went along. I didn't understand why Winnie permanently moved slowly at a snail's pace. Winnie was disoriented when she used the walker. Now rethinking, that was a symptom of Alzheimer's. My son Pat, an MD, suggested I start a regimen of vitamins for his grandmother. He had found it helpful in some situations. I tried, but Winnie wouldn't take them unless I stood there and watched her. Sometimes she would spit them out, claiming I was trying to poison her. She had no interest in helping herself and would not listen when I tried to explain why I wanted her to take vitamins.

She wouldn't come to the farmhouse for meals. But, on the other hand, she wouldn't eat unless Jim or I sat with her at her house. After the loss of Rusty, we had another dog. If we weren't looking, she fed her food to Bo (a Chesapeake Bay Retriever). An interesting sideline, the dog, didn't like anybody except Jim (his dog) or me because I fed her when Jim was at work. But Bo fell in love with Jim's mother. She would lie on the porch and watch the driveway and the property from every direction, guard dog extraordinary. On one sweltering day, I went over to Winnie's to check on her, and Bo was under a throw rug, panting. I asked Winnie why Bo was under the rug, and she said, "Bo was cold, so I wanted to keep her warm. She was shivering, and I knew she was cold." Bo would put up with anything Winnie did. Unbelievable.

One Saturday, I had a meeting in Helena and would be gone overnight. Jim was at work, so I took two bowls of dog food over to Winnie and asked if she would feed Bo her supper and breakfast while I was gone. She went into a rage. "I'm not eating dog food. Are you trying to poison me? I'm not eating dog food." I tried to explain it was for Bo while I was in Helena for a meeting. She went into another rant, screaming about not eating dog food.

After her arguing got more and more heated, I finally told her I had to leave. I called Hugh, a long-time friend, to ask if he would check on Winnie because she was in such a state. I told him she would probably yell and carry on and that he should be aware. When I returned the next day and called him to see how it went, he said she couldn't have been more pleasant. They went to dinner, and he fed Bo, and everything worked out fine.

The Saturday episode was one of the indications she was having memory problems and the other disturbing signals. She started throwing things in the garbage, pictures, cans of food, and bread, and I don't know what else before discovering what she was doing. She put her silverware in the refrigerator and threw tomatoes and eggs into the trash. The loaves of bread she didn't feed Bo she threw into the garbage. I searched every day. I didn't know from one day to the next what I would find. I asked her to stop throwing pictures in the trash. She insisted nobody wanted them, so I continued the retrieval. Winnie refused to close her door, and there was a mouse invasion when the weather changed. Jim installed an automatic closer, which worked, but she incessantly complained that we were locking her in. Nonsense, of course.

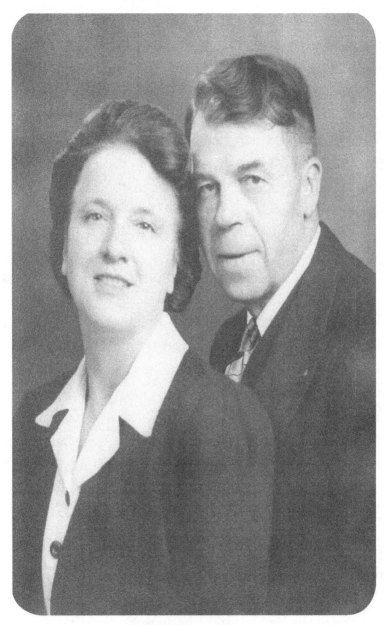

Winnifred and Jay

With Jim's mother living at the farm, it was almost a daily intervention between them if he wasn't on a run (railroad jargon) on the Railroad. They were at odds about everything. She accused him of not caring about her, and he accused her of being bossy and overbearing. On other days she was as sweet as pie, and if he was having a good day, they got along great. But I never knew which personality would be dominant on any particular day. It was stressful and nerve-racking. Thinking back on it now, I think Winnie was in the middle stages of Alzheimer's. In my observation, I believe the tendency toward the condition might be hereditary. Research is leaning in that direction as well, although brain injuries are probably the principal reason.

Winnie was a very generous person. If she had a visitor, she always had cookies or cake, something to serve. For my birthday, Winnifred made ginger cream cookies with powder sugar frosting because they were my favorite. We were friends, and I think if Jim and I ever had a dispute of some kind, she would have taken my side. I grew to love her, even the crankiness and obstinate disagreements. Winnifred wouldn't accept thanks for anything; she brushed it aside. I think she was probably embarrassed if anyone praised her.

Chris, Jim's cousin, and Earl stopped one afternoon to see Winnie. Chris commented to me that Winnie didn't have any food in her refrigerator. I explained that I had stocked her frig and cupboard the day before. I hadn't checked that day, so she had probably thrown everything into the trash. Chris asked what they could do. There was nothing since they lived in Lake Stevens, Washington, at that time.

Life went smoothly for a couple of months. Our son, Jan,

his wife, and some friends, including Hugh, stopped by in early August. They spent time with Winnie and had an extended visit, reminiscing, and she was relaxed and talkative. They left about two o'clock, and I went over to the trailer at four-thirty to take her dinner. Winnie was lying on the floor by the sofa. I tried to help her up, but she was a deadweight. I couldn't lift her, so I pushed her into a sitting position. After struggling for several minutes, I tried to explain that I could push her up onto the sofa if she could get onto her knees. But, she was so disoriented; she couldn't understand what I wanted her to do. After a half-hour of trying to help her, I was exhausted and thought I should call her doctor.

The doctor told me Winnie might have hurt her back, and I should call an ambulance and take her to the hospital. He would meet me there. She was finally calm and asked what was happening. I told her I talked with the doctor, and he wanted to examine her. I put Bo in the house. I wasn't sure how she would react when the medics arrived. She was so protective of Winnie. Reaching the hospital, Winnie said she was cold, so I located a nurse and got a blanket. We waited a while for the doctor, and Winnie wanted to know why she was there and could she go home. I reminded Winnie she had fallen, and the doctor wanted to be sure she was okay but asked again a few minutes later.

She spent two days in the hospital. The doctor moved her to an extended care facility attached to the hospital. The doctor explained that she needed to gain some strength, and with therapy, she could go home in a few days. But, being obstinate, she wouldn't cooperate and complained nonstop. Jim and I joined her for lunch at the facility a few times. She complained about the food, she complained about her room, she complained it was too hot or too cold. She complained if we visited, and the nurse said she complained that we hadn't come to visit.

Over the course of the month, she began to deteriorate. She decided that she wouldn't eat and clamped her mouth so the nurse couldn't feed her. We consulted with the doctor. He said he could put her on a regimen to help her regain strength and mobility, but she would be right back in the same situation as soon as it stopped.

Jim called his sister to ask her opinion of what to do. Shirley drove over from Spokane to meet with the doctor, Jim, and me. Shirley and Jim agreed to follow the doctor's advice about their mother and not intervene. Winnie continued to refuse to eat. Every visit, she repeated she wanted to die, to me and to anyone who would listen. Winnie stated, over and over, that all her friends were already dead and didn't want to live. I continued to say we cared about her, but she said she didn't have a reason to live. I explained again and again that we wanted her alive. Winnie didn't want to get out of bed and repeated over and over, "Just let me die, please, let me die." The nurses and the doctor couldn't force her to eat, and I couldn't convince her either. I watched this beautiful woman wither and decline. She died three weeks later. It was heartrending and sad to see a once vibrant, delightful lady waste away. She was a shell of her former self.

The funeral home was overflowing with flowers. She belonged to the Rebecka's Organization for years, and the women held a small service within the funeral service. People told me stories about how they met her and how they enjoyed her. She was much loved and didn't seem to know it. For most of her life, Winnie had been cantankerous and obstinate. She wouldn't accept thanks for anything she did for anyone. It didn't surprise me that so many people cared about her.

Following Winnie's death, it took time to settle into any sort of routine. We sold the trailer, and I had to decide what to do with her personal belongings. She didn't leave a will, and I had no idea what she might want to have done with anything she owned. Jim's sister helped sort out a few things she thought people might want, such as pictures or silverware. I put most of it into our storage and included a few items to donate to the Salvation Army. She had already thrown away most of her possessions during the summer. I kept a vase that had been in her family for a long time. She had a lamp she was fond of, and I asked Shirley if she wanted it. When Shirley said no, I gave it to the people who bought the trailer.

We were adjusting to the emptiness. I hadn't realized how much of our lives Winnie occupied. Bo looked for her for weeks. Now and then, I would start to fix a tray for her, which would strike me that it wasn't necessary.

The farm continued to be a haven from the troubles, anxieties, and tribulations of work issues and the increasing memory loss incidents. They were coming more often, and the paranoia seemed more extreme and lasted longer. Nevertheless, they were still far enough apart that I could push them away temporarily. It was easy to rationalize that nothing was really wrong.

I was running for reelection to the State Legislature in 1988. Meanwhile, the Flathead County Central Committee elected me as a delegate for Dukakis. I attended the National Democratic Convention held in Atlanta, Georgia. Jean, my campaign treasurer, accompanied me. Unaccustomed to the humidity, my feet swelled so much I had to buy shoes, which was a weird experience I had never encountered living in Montana. Of course, when I returned home, the shoes were too big. I think I gave them to charity since they were new.

The state chairman gave me tickets to the Reporters' reception, held on the CNN center's upper floor on Sunday morning. We had our picture taken with all sorts of celebrities, such as Tom Brokaw, Peter Jennings, Sander Vanoker, and Ted Koppel.

Senator Max Baucus hosted a Governor's farewell cocktail party for retiring Montana Governor Ted Schwinden. It was heart-warming to see the friendly affection held toward our Governor. William (Bill} Clinton was the Governor of Arkansas at the time. The affair was on the seventh floor, with floor-to-ceiling windows. The city view was spectacular, but we congregated in the opposite area, away from the glass. It was scary to be looking out with only a glass wall between us and the street below. It was a sickening feeling. Someone closed the drapes and thus eliminated the anxiety.

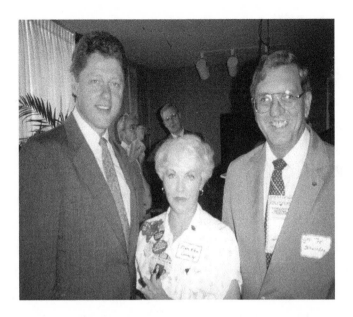

President Clinton, Mary Ellen, Governor Schwinden

Nine

When Jim retired, we settled into a more ordinary routine. Although I still had to attend meetings and the regular sessions of the Legislature. The episodes were still few and far between, and I had the feeling we should do a few of the things we had planned for retirement. We spent a week in Italy on the Italian Riviera and a week in Spain visiting the attractions and experimenting with local food. The restaurants in Spain served salads like a work of art. They were truly spectacular with patterns and colors. Jim loved the salads. The olive trees in Spain were very different from the olive trees in Italy. I had a fleeting moment, wondering why. Lovely little towns with narrow streets and cobblestones. The clerk spoke a smattering of English in most stores, so we didn't have language differences.

We rented a car and toured the area, the Leaning tower in Italy. We sat for a while at Piza, and four teenage girls came over and talked with us. They each had different colored hair, bright red, orange, green, and purple. They knew we were from the states, I guess. They asked if they could sit with us. I was surprised how well they spoke English, although with a very definite accent. They wanted to know about the United States. Everybody knew California, but when we said we were from Montana, they wanted to know where it was. They weren't aware of the different states, thinking California was the totality of our country. We had a problem explaining, and they asked lots of questions. I spent time learning the language, so I used my guidebook a lot, but they were pretty impressive. I asked to take their picture, and they agreed, and they took our picture. The girls asked me to write our names. When I think about those girls, it occurred to me; I didn't get their names. It would have been fun to write and stay in touch.

Driving in Italy is the most frightening thing I experienced. They drove 90 miles an hour, no matter whether on a city street, a road, or the Audubon. The streets in the small towns weren't as wide as our alleys. The Italians drove up on the sidewalk to pass. We were there three days before we discovered huge mirrors at the intersections. I suspect that's why they drove like crazy. Jim was beginning to operate the same way, and that was frightening. Scooters charged in and out of traffic. Strangely with all the undisciplined driving, we didn't see an accident. The only time we spotted an officer was when they stopped a pretty girl with no sign of a ticket book. Just to chat, I guess.

While driving in Rome, we searched for a specific museum, but we couldn't find the street. With eight lanes of traffic, we decided to pull over to a side street. But I couldn't make sense of the map, so I went into a tiny tobacco store to ask for directions. The clerk didn't speak English. He called his wife from a back room. She understood only a few words, so I pointed to the listing in the guidebook. The door opened, and a man came in to ask what was going on. The door opened again, and two men came in. Everybody was talking at once, and I couldn't explain what I wanted to know. Another man came in, and I decided nothing was going to help. When I left the shop, they were still waving arms, gesturing, and arguing at the top of their voices. I didn't have a clue what they were saying. We found the museum, but only by accident. We had to cross six lanes of traffic, which was hairraising, and we held our breath until we made it across. Quite often traffic lights were not working.

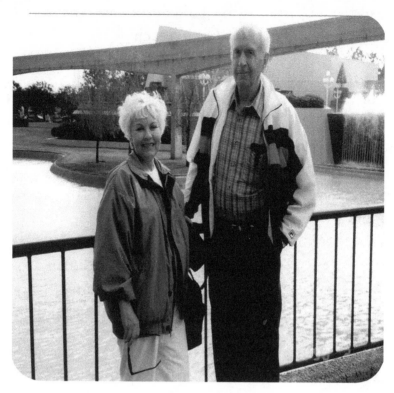

Jum & Muz - Italy

In 1995 we rented an apartment with two friends and lived in Paris for a month. The apartment was in a residential area. There was a farmer's market every morning at ten, and the street department washed the streets at six using Fire hoses. Everyone had a dog (sometimes two or three), and they pooped everywhere, so I assume that was the reason for the washing. It certainly solved the poop problem. The apartment had a tiny washing machine and metered the electricity. I figured out the controls, so I did everyone's laundry.

Several restaurants were close to the apartment. Small shops and a supermarket were also in the area. In the market, everything was on open shelves, and there was no refrigeration. We did not buy milk, but if you bought a loaf of bread or something of that sort, it was placed inside a sheet of paper.

No sacks and quite rudimentary compared to the U. S. supermarkets. They had a fabulous wine collection, however.

We took a train to Normandy, rented a car, and toured the allied D-Day invasion's five beaches. Artillery and rusted-out equipment, abandoned when the conflict ended, remain a grim reminder of the carnage. The War museum on the site depicted the history of the battle. We were quiet as we moved from one beach to another of the five beaches. I thought of the totality of the courage shown by the men involved.

We searched the American cemetery with our friend looking for her nephew, killed during the conflict. Acres of white crosses put a catch in your throat. Jim was unusually quiet, and I wondered if he remembered his experience during the war. It was heart-breaking, walking through the memories of that dreadful day. The cemetery reminded me that my Aunt Hulda had a grandson killed and was MIA. She died before I could find out if he had been found.

Returning to Paris, Jim was confused at the apartment complex and couldn't remember where we had to go. I took his hand, and he didn't question where we were.

Jim and I attended a production and dinner at the Moulin Rouge. A truly spectacular performance. The table seated eight, and we each introduced ourselves. A couple from Japan kept falling asleep. They were suffering jet-lag and missed large parts of the show. Of course, we toured the castles and dungeons and prisons that everyone visits. We had a curious experience when we went to dinner at the restaurant at the top of the East India Museum. Carlotta, our friend, had her fork on the way to her mouth when the waiter took her plate. We had not finished our meal, but they hustled us out. I guess it's true; the wait staff doesn't like the ugly Americans. We were not impressed, definitely disappointed, and the food wasn't all that good, either.

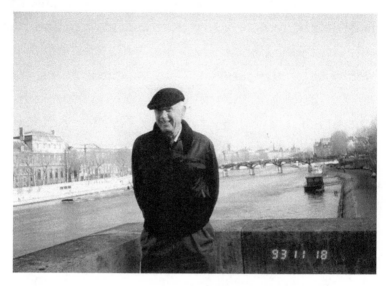

Jum – Paris 1993

We took two trips to Mexico with my sister Helen and her husband Albert, nickname Abby. Fun trips without a sign of confusion and bewilderment from Jim. On our first trip, the power went off for two days at the resort. We decided to move to an international hotel with backup power. But it was OK because there was a vast pool complex with a swim-up bar. We lazed and sipped drinks for the remainder of the trip. Every afternoon at four, it began to rain. Within an hour, the water was a foot deep along the streets, continuing for two hours, and stopped abruptly. The following day there was no sign of the water. On schedule, at four, the rain began again and continued the two weeks of our stay. We had dinner at a tiny restaurant where the front entrance had stands of parrots. They were every color, some huge and some very small. I wondered how the owner kept them on the various perches since they were not in cages.

We were so close to the water waves were lapping against the deck on the second trip to Puerto Vallarta. We rented a fishing boat for a day. Jim and Abby caught a sailfish in the first half-hour. I felt a pull on my line, and the captain yelled, "reel him in, reel him in." I wound the reel, and forty-five minutes passed, and I still didn't have the fish in the boat.

As a fish jumped several hundred feet from the boat, I yelled, "Look, there's another fish." Jim laughed and said, "That's your fish." I hadn't moved him at all. Jim helped me reel, and finally, the sailfish was in the boat. Helen also had a fish take her line but lost it. The captain said we had to go back because we had three fish. Our boat won the daily prize for the most fish.

The guy at the dock kidded Jim and me about being newlyweds and gave us 'two for the price of one,' to have them mounted and shipped to us. Abby was a little peeved because he paid for one at the same price, Jim and I paid for two. I was a little concerned we wouldn't see the fish again. But about six months later, they arrived at the Port at Butte, Montana. We had to bail them out, and I found a guy driving to Kalispell, and he delivered our fish.

The third trip with Helen and Abby was three weeks in the UK. We spent a week in England, a week in Ireland, and a week in Scotland. It was an excruciating experience driving on the left side of the road. Jim had a few days of confusion, and the Emphysema was giving him trouble with walking. He had to stop often, no matter if we only walked a short distance.

Arriving at Heathrow Airport, we rented a car. But then, the dilemma of who would drive. We decided to draw names for only one person to do that, and Abby won the draw. But we were petrified. Consequently, we were incessantly yelling at him to stay left. He was a good sport. We probably caused him headaches by our paranoid screaming.

We stayed in a castle where Shakespeare wrote his plays at Stratford on Avon in England. The rooms we occupied were in a converted stable. Acres of green lawn surrounded the area. We watched the changing of the guard at Windsor Castle. Big Ben was closed off for cleaning, so construction blocked some of the streets. But, we walked everywhere and saved Abby from too much stress driving.

Ireland was the greenest green you can imagine. It's greener than green, if that makes sense. We stayed in a bed and breakfast, but the breakfasts were enough for ten people. There was no central heating. The bedrooms had gorgeous quilts, so heavy they made your legs ache. Jim said we must not go to Northern Ireland. Abby asked why, and Jim answered," because the government might arrest him." His relatives were from the north, "Pig under the Bed Irish," his dad had told him. We weren't sure if this was true, but it was a good story.

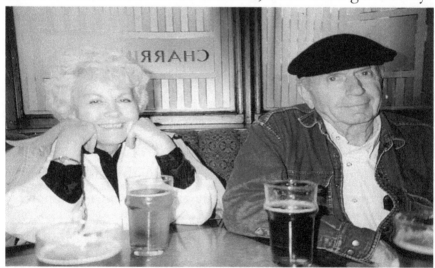

Jum & Muz   Ireland – 1995

The Irish pub had a huge sign that said, 'no singing allowed.' I thought this very odd. How could you not sing along with the incredible music? I wondered what would happen if they caught you singing. The Irish have countless rousing and memorable songs built for singing. The melancholy sadness that permeates Ireland made me feel sad.

Scotland was the most laid-back and relaxed. The pub at the resort had live music every night. There was only one minor incident at the resort. Jim didn't want to go with us one night to listen to music. We started back to our rooms an hour later, and Jim stood by the pub's front door. He didn't know why or how long he had been there. He was okay for the remainder of our stay and the trip home.

Abby developed unrelenting headaches. We thought it was probably the stress of the left side of the road driving. We talked about the change to the left-side and decided to draw names for a designated driver, and Abby won or lost if you look at it that way. We thought it would probably be better because of the pressure if one person did all the driving. We spent a great deal of time yelling and reminding him, which undoubtedly contributed to the headaches. Helen convinced him to see a doctor, and he received medication. The doctor told him to be sure to get checked out at home, which he did.

Returning home, it was becoming more noticeable that Jim didn't remember everyday occurrences. He wasn't sure how to use a toothbrush. He paced, back and forth from the living room to the kitchen and back to the living room. When the toilet plugged up, Jim put a sign on the door – 'out of order.' – He didn't know how to fix it and was confused as to why it wouldn't flush, continually asking over and over, "Why won't it work?" Just small things, but very frustrating and upsetting to him, and also disturbing to me. I had to be aware every waking moment, at any time, of some unforeseen incident. Probably the first occurrence was while we were still on the farm. Jim could not find the post office. He asked," when it had moved because it wasn't where it was supposed to be?" He began continually asking where I had parked the car. I always told him it was by the house, where it was parked all the time. But he continued to ask.

In the later years, Jim slept only a few hours at one time and wandered during the night, another cause for worry. I wasn't getting enough sleep because he woke me when he got out of bed. I couldn't be sure if he had to go to the bathroom or just wander. Occasionally, I could convince him to return to bed, but sometimes not, depending on the time. If it was 2 or 3 in the morning, he wanted to move to the sofa to sleep, but never longer than a few hours. The restlessness grew worse as time passed, and the pacing was continuous on some days. I was at my wit's end. I wasn't getting any sleep, and I was beginning to think I would never get any sleep. It wears you down. You are exhausted, with no end in sight.

When Trace, our grandson, was being married, we took the train to Wisconsin. Following the reception, we returned to the hotel around ten. I was removing the bedspread, and Jim somehow unfastened the security lock on the door and disappeared. I called the desk, and the clerk said he would search. I looked up and down the hallways without finding him. I checked back at the room, and he was not there. As I was going down the hall again, he emerged from the elevator. I do not know where he had been, and he couldn't remember. The desk clerk said he hadn't seen him. I locked the door again, placing a chair against it, but slept fitfully. I could not be sure he wouldn't disappear, and I would not be able to find him. The following day he had no memory of the night before.

The plane ride home was uneventful, although Jim questioned why the meal delivery took so long. He was becoming agitated when the food arrived. If we went to a restaurant, Jim couldn't relax while we waited. He would begin to fidget, asking over and over what was taking so long, even if it had been only a few minutes. I decided it wasn't worth the hassle, and we did not go out to eat unless I had someone with us or it was a special occasion.

One year Pat and his family were in Yellowstone Park, and Becki, Mike, Jim, and I planned to meet them. Connections were lousy, and we flew to Idaho Falls and drove to Jackson Hole, Wyoming. I rented a timeshare, and it was a short trip to the Park. While I was checking in, Jim took off down the road, and Mike ran after him. He said he had to talk and talk to persuade his Grampa to come back. It was frustrating trying to keep track of him. Another frustrating symptom of Alzheimer's is the tendency to wander with no idea where they might be going.

The next day, waiting to hear from Pat, we decided to take the tram to the top of a mountain vista area. We had been there only a half-hour when the attendant told us we had to go down because of the threat of lightning and thunderstorms. We were waiting inside the wheelhouse when it started to rain. Three people were outside when the first car stopped, and they boarded. Jim charged out before we could stop him, climbed into the car, and left to go down the mountain. We had to wait for the next one (about fifteen minutes). We talked to each other, worrying whether Jim would be gone, and we would never find him. But, lo and behold, when we reached the bottom, he was sitting on a bench, waiting. We all gave a huge sigh of relief.

We drove to the Park to meet Pat and his family. We watched Old Faithful perform, and following the spectacular geyser, walked back to the Lodge for lunch. We stood by the front entrance waiting for the throng of tourists to thin out as they formed a line loading a bus. Jim suddenly went over and joined the line of people getting on the bus. Pat noticed him just as he climbed the step. Luckily he grabbed him in time, or he could have been long gone. After that, we took turns, so someone watched him at all times. He was so swift and agile he could be gone in a couple of minutes.

The park personnel presented programs at various times. Following lunch, we were standing in a circle watching a Cowboy twirling a rope and giving a spiel about the Wild West. He asked if anyone was from Canada, and Jim spoke up and said yes, he was. The Cowboy told a joke and then asked if anyone was there from New York, and Jim spoke up and said he was. The guy laughed and made a silly joke, and of course, the crowd joined in the laugher. The kids were embarrassed, but Pat explained to them it was all in good fun. Probably the group thought Jim was a plant as part of the act. We had a great time; the kids saw a moose, an elk, and several bears. The ranger told us most of the bears had been moved out of the area because tourists were feeding them, and they had become very aggressive and a hazard.

The trip home was unexciting. Life returned to a semi-normal atmosphere, about as typical as possible with the continuing anxiety and Jim's increasing frustration. Anxiety can become very debilitating, and I found myself trying to rationalize all the time. That was frustrating in itself.

As a family, we planned a day-long trip through and north of the San Juan Islands. News reports stated whales were seen in the area at that time of year. As we traveled through the islands, the boat circled, and the captain said he would call out if he spotted a whale. Jan's wife, Minde, brought lunch, and we had snacks and jackets if the weather turned cold or windy. Two other groups were on the same trip, and each group provided their cooler. When lunchtime arrived, Minde handed out sandwiches and drinks.

Apparently, Jim decided to check out the other coolers, because Mike caught him just as he started to open one. Mike apologized to the people with a silly explanation, and we had a good laugh. Sad to say, we didn't see a whale after all. But the scenery was spectacular, the trip was fun, and we enjoyed the day. It turned out to be one of the last trips we took together as a family.

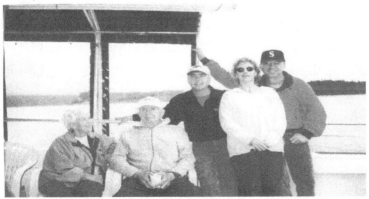

Whale Watching
Mary Ellen, Jim, Pat, Becki, Jan

Ten

In 1992 we listed the farm for sale. My final term in the Legislature would end in December, and we decided to move to the Seattle area. We were tired of the ice and snow of Montana. It made sense to be closer to Becki and her family. That summer became an incredible, unbelievable nightmare.

The Governor called a special session of the Legislature in July. But, I had been elected a delegate and was attending the Democratic Convention in New York City. After the convention, I returned from New York City to join the legislature in Helena. I called my husband to tell him I was back in Montana. The session, scheduled to end the next day, was Saturday. Jim told me he had just hung up the phone after a call from our son, Pat. Our granddaughter Tara was with another girl, and they were riding a jet ski. They were going too fast, and a sharp turn threw Tara against a concrete wall and killed her instantly. A senseless boating accident in Wisconsin.

Tara was eight, and her brother Trace was eleven when Pat and their mother married. Pat was completing his OB/GYN specialty at the University at Madison. We met the children at the wedding and were friends immediately. We welcomed them into our family.

Tara and I hit it off from the start. During the six days we spent there, we discovered mutual interests, and she became my soulmate. We both loved clothes, and Tara insisted I must look at a specialty shop. She was right. It was a great afternoon of shopping. She had thick blond hair, and I asked if she wanted me to show her how to French braid. She agreed instantly, and we had another way to communicate as friends. On subsequent visits, she woke me every morning to braid her hair before school.

Visiting back and forth the next few years, Trace and I became friends as well. He was a fanatic golfer, and Jim liked to golf, so they had long talks about golf and baseball. Ryan and Caitlin were born into the family, and Trace loved to babysit. Tara was fifteen when she died; a fluke, a senseless accident on a jet-ski. The family was in total desolation. She left a vacuum no one could fill. I felt equally at a loss because we had become close. Losing a child is so incredibly painful and such a waste, a lovely young girl with her whole life before her.

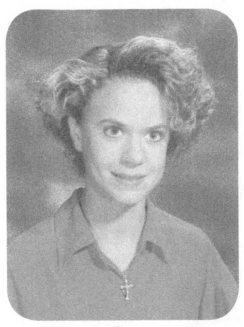

Tara

In addition to that horrible news, my sister (Vera Mae) Babe called to tell me our mother was failing rapidly. Mom had suffered a stroke the previous December and was bed-ridden. Babe cared for her with the help of a visiting nurse during the week. A few years earlier, after her husband died, Babe offered to have Mom live with her. Mom could no longer live alone because of failing eyesight. Evelyn and her husband, Bob, had four acres near Fortine, Montana. They suggested Babe move a trailer house to their property. Later, Dorothy bought a trailer, and it was moved to the four acres, as well.

After Bob died, my sisters, Evelyn, Babe, and Dorothy, lived in the three-way complex they had developed, and each sister had their own home. I made the forty-mile trip to Fortine at least once a week. But, nothing changed in my mother's condition over the months. The doctor said our mother's chances for recovery were slim, and he recommended ways to make her comfortable. Babe said she would keep me in touch with whatever was happening, if our mother's condition improved, or if anything changed.

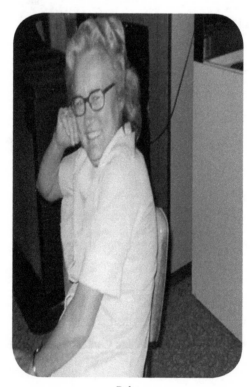

Babe

In July, while dealing with those troubling circumstances, we had an offer on the property. We hesitated whether to go ahead. I had qualms of whether I wanted to deal with the sale and moving and Jim's problems. We discussed it at length, trying to make a decision that made sense. Nevertheless, despite all that happened, we began the process of negotiating the paperwork.

We met with the Real Estate Agent; she presented and discussed the proposal offered on the farmhouse and ten acres. Agents from a different office brought an offer on the raw acreage, and they left paperwork with us. We discussed with our agent the best way to accommodate the two separate proposals. We considered changing the ten-acre parcel's direction from north-south to east-west to adjust for the other offer if acceptable to both parties. The agent said she would get back to us with the possible changes. The proposed sale became a nightmare before anything had been settled or finalized.

The agent brought the paperwork for the changes. I wanted to review them, but she pressured us to agree to other changes during the acreage division. She inadvertently revealed she had never handled a sale of a complicated property. She had only dealt with single-family homes. We hired a lawyer to clarify the paperwork and straighten out the differences.

The lawyer told us we should try to settle and sign their agreement. I refused and kept refusing until worn down emotionally. Jim was having anxiety attacks caused by continual arguing and pressure from the agent and the lawyer. I felt as though I was falling apart. My stomach hurt, and I couldn't sleep. Meanwhile, the agent and the lawyer continued to hassle us to make a decision.

Following a survey, the property was in the process of being divided into two parcels. A smaller tract contained ten acres, the house, barn, chicken coop, and two out-buildings. The other tract consisted of 40 acres of raw land. The survey was not consistent with the plat description, confusing the issue. I walked the property line with the buyers interested in the 10 acres to show them approximately how the 10 acres would appear in the new direction. The walkthrough happened before I found a discrepancy in the size of the parcel. It turned out there was an extra 3 acres, now in dispute, not listed in the original agreement as part of the 10-acre piece. The second buyer wanted only thirty-four acres. The three in the discrepancy would be left in limbo because there would not be access to the parcel.

The Realtor told me we had to give the buyers the other 3 acres. They now owned it psychologically because I had pointed it out to them. I had not. Finally, after another late-night session with the lawyer, the agent agreed to forego her commission to cover 2 acres. The buyers would finance the other acre. The agent signed the statement as she agreed.

The survey was taking longer than anticipated. Meanwhile, our lawyer presented an agreement for us to move by the 17th of September. I'm not sure why this became a priority since we had not transferred the title or received any money. However, we thought he knew what he was doing. The buyers of the ten acres had sold their house and had to move. I wondered why this became our problem, and the lawyer did not explain. I was under such pressure that I did not pursue it. It became apparent that I should have demanded an explanation.

We began moving stuff into a rental. The potential

buyers agreed we could store boxes on the front porch of the farmhouse. We needed more time to take them to storage or charity because we took other items to the rental.

Meanwhile, I was trying to stay calm and not fall apart. My nephew was helping with the transfer of a freezer to the rental. Jim told him to wait for the signal to lift the shell to remove it. The bed had to be open to allow enough room to load the freezer. Just as he said that, my nephew shoved it, it tilted, striking Jim in the head. He suffered a gash requiring eleven stitches. I was worried about the meat in the freezer thawing out, which was ridiculous.

After they loaded the freezer, I told Jim to drive himself to the emergency. He was bleeding profusely by that time, and I handed him a towel for his head. I was distraught, and I wasn't thinking. My god, he probably had a concussion. I'm not even sure Jim would have known where to find the emergency room. Just one more example of the pressure we were experiencing. Without question, ridiculous incidents kept happening. Having to deal with them contributed to our increasing anxiety and distress. The realtor phoned with new items to discuss. She wanted to know why nothing was progressing on schedule, and it must be my fault.   Why else?

During the fiasco of the property sale, my mother suffered a further setback from the stroke and was in serious condition. I was driving back and forth every other day to be with her. Besides, we were packing boxes and sorting items. My mother was at my sister's in Fortine, which is approximately 40 miles from the farm. Babe said I should prepare for the worst.

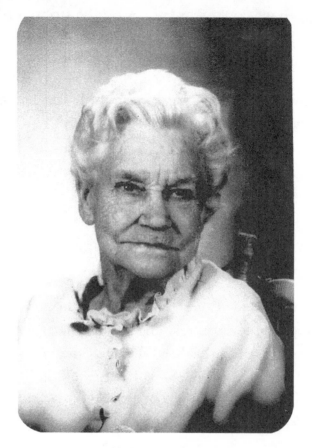

My Mom – Esther

My mother died on a Tuesday in September. There was a Memorial service in Eureka for Friday and buried in Sandpoint, Idaho, the following Monday. The Buyers wanted to move into the farmhouse on Friday. We couldn't be available because of the memorial and pending funeral. Our daughter arrived from Seattle to be at the services of her grandmother. Meanwhile, we fired the original lawyer and hired a different lawyer to organize and, if possible, save us from more entanglements

Thursday, the Realtor came to the rental to ask for a key to the farmhouse. She insisted she would be there on Friday. The buyers were still planning to move into the house on Friday. Even though I had explained, we were committed to the memorial and funeral of my mother. The agent said she would oversee the buyers moving our remaining items to the porch. I didn't want them to have permission but finally agreed. I was so exhausted that I just wanted her to go away and leave me alone.

Early Friday morning, Jim went to the farmhouse to move our finished boxes to the porch. It was getting toward noon, and he had not returned, so Becki and I took his suit and tie and drove to the farm. We were running late to the memorial, and we had to leave Bo at the house. There was no time to take her back to the rental.

The buyers turned up at the house, and Bo wouldn't let them in. They complained to the Realtor that we had done that on purpose. She called and would not listen when we tried to explain leaving the dog. The three of us, Becki, Jim, and I, were tired and upset. The weekend became even more of a disaster.

When we arrived to move boxes, the buyers were in the house Saturday morning with several other people. I sorted papers and legislative reports into two separate stacks for donating to the library and my records. The buyers had thrown everything into a single pile, thus negating three months' work. They pushed boxes together, mixing those for the Salvation Army with ours. I didn't know which boxes were which. I hadn't marked them. They threw a pile of trash into the legislative papers designated for the Library. I was outraged. I was angry and upset. My daughter told the people they had to leave immediately.

The agent had promised she would be there. However, when we arrived on Saturday, she was nowhere to be found. I should have called the Sheriff and had the buyers removed from the property. When the telephone rang, I answered, and the wife wanted to know why I was answering her phone. She tried to speak to her husband, and I hung up. I did not want to talk with her.

Still arguing they had a right to be there, the buyers left. We tried to sort out the disarray of the boxes, the papers, and the trash. I was utterly discouraged. Becki and Jim were equally upset, but they tried to console me. Furthermore, I was concerned that the stress and pressure on Jim might trigger an episode. To my relief, that didn't happen.

We had just come back from the memorial for my mother. We still planned to drive to Sandpoint for the funeral service scheduled for Monday afternoon. My mother had been ill for ten months, but I still wasn't prepared to deal with her death at age ninety-six. I was trying to hold myself together for my sanity but also for Jim and the rest of my family.

On Saturday, I had asked the buyer (a pastor of a local church), "don't you have compassion for our situation with the death of my mother?" He told me he had plenty of compassion, but a contract was a contract. So much for so-called Christian charity.

Monday morning, my niece, Donna, offered her van to drive my three sisters, Becki and me, to Sandpoint for Mom's funeral. Jim stated he didn't want to ride with us; he would take his pickup because he wanted to take Bo along. Following the funeral, we were at the reception at the home of my sister Charlotte. Jim said he was leaving to go back to Montana. He was adamant that he leave immediately. I didn't want to argue in front of everyone, so I agreed. I was apprehensive that he would make it back without getting lost. However, he drove to Sandpoint by himself, so I had to take that chance. He was safe at home when we arrived at the rental that evening. I can't explain the feeling of relief.

Tuesday morning, we still had to deal with property problems; the cost, extra expense, and stress. The original lawyer divulged later that he had never done any real estate work. That became obvious as the months passed, and everything was getting screwed up. He also told us he hadn't done very well by us. The lawyer cost us dearly. Especially his insistence that we had to move. We signed the agreement before the title company completed the paperwork for the sale. I have never understood the reasoning of the lawyer in that respect. His rationale was that the buyers of the farmhouse had sold their house and had to move early. How was that our problem? Ignorance was in abundance. With the continual conflict, we were stressed and anxious. I'm not sure we were thinking straight, and indeed, we depended too much on the lawyer's advice, which turned out to be wrong and against our interests.

A week before their scheduled move into the farmhouse, I called the buyers to ask if they were interested in meeting for details of the many idiosyncrasies of an old house. The Pastor told me, "No, we aren't interested." Instead, he called their lawyer, who met with our lawyer. Whatever the discussion at that meeting, there is no doubt it wasn't to our benefit.

I was upset, distraught, worried, and unable to sleep, trying to cope with the agent and the lawyer. We ended up moving before the title transfer, paying rent for three months and the extra insurance by the forced move. The lawyers, the agent, and the buyers together created the turmoil. It was an ordeal from the beginning.

There was never a meeting of the minds and never a resolution of the conflict. Never an attempt to step back or any attempt to tell us this was not going to work. There was no mention of a mistake, and we should start over. The upheaval in our lives lasted five months, but the distress and bad feelings will take a long time for full recovery – maybe never. A friend of ours, a judge, told me we should have taken them to court to settle the dispute, if only on principle. We would have won.

I also wonder how much of the disorder and commotion accelerated the memory confusion in Jim. Knowing the effect on me, I'm confident that the stress must have affected Jim with the disruption it caused in our lives. Likely, the agent and the lawyers are still causing problems with their lack of integrity and incompetence. The people who bought the farmhouse have since sold and moved. I guess they found out they should have accepted my offer to explain the eccentricities of an old house.

Eleven

Packing for the move to the coast, we were doing the follow-up necessary to tie up loose ends. I had a scheduled doctor appointment, and a December mammogram uncovered a lump in my breast. Following a biopsy, a tumor diagnosis, I had a lumpectomy. Following the surgery, we moved to Washington state. Eight weeks of radiation would take place in Everett, Washington, at the cancer center. The treatment was successful and determined that I was cancer-free.

My term in the House of Representatives expired at the end of the year, and we were packed and ready. Finally, in December, we were moving to Mukilteo, Washington. I couldn't drive because of the surgery. Becki flew back to drive my car, packed with household items. Jim followed in the pickup. We cautioned Jim to follow close behind us. I was concerned he might get lost if he became disoriented as he drove with Bo and a load. However, he did okay, but we kept him in sight in the rear-view mirror, just in case. We spent the night with Jim's sister in Spokane. Jim plugged the freezer into her garage outlet. We left early to fill the gas tanks and checked to keep Jim with us while we maneuvered through side streets.

The dog was twelve and couldn't jump up to the seat any longer, so Jim had built a set of steps to help her. In the preparations for the move, he tied the steps to the top of the pickup. The freezer was in the back and loaded to the roof, and my Blazer also packed solid. A friend of Becki's met the movers since we would be late arriving. The alarm was blaring, and she had to dismantle it because the power had been off, and the code wouldn't work. Becki commented that we looked like Montana hippies or hillbillies. I wonder what the folks in Mukilteo thought when they had that first glimpse of us. But they waved and were friendly.

A little girl across the street brought cookies a few days after we moved in. She stated that her mother said, "welcome." One day I heard the girl talking with a friend, as she mentioned her new neighbor must be really, really old because her hair was white. I had to laugh. Pretty observant; she was four and talked a mile a minute.

During the move to Mukilteo, we stopped overnight with Shirley. She didn't seem to be her usual self, and I commented to Becki. She agreed that Shirley seemed vague, with silence when usually talkative. She took forever to fix breakfast. I asked the location of the nearest gas station, Shirley couldn't explain how to get there. She couldn't remember the streets or the name of the station. She gave us the general direction of a station, and we found it eventually.

She responded with hugs when we were leaving. Although we noticed she was quiet and more restrained than usual, I was not convinced of an actual change in her behavior. I telephoned Shirley now and then after we moved, and she seemed to be alert and with it.

In 1996 our granddaughter (Jan's daughter) was married in Spokane, and we attended the wedding. Shirley was very frail and didn't respond readily. At the reception, we sat with Shirley and Jim's niece, Connie. Shirley sat silently. If we asked a question, she answered. Her words were slow, and she struggled to express them. I commented to Becki that something was definitely wrong and. Becki agreed. They left early, which was very unusual. Ordinarily, Shirley would have enjoyed the music and spent time visiting.

Several years later, when Shirley died, we drove to Spokane for the funeral. Following the service in a conversation, her best friend told me Shirley had Alzheimer's. I had suspected it because she had all the symptoms Jim had exhibited. I didn't see her often, but Shirley was more vague, withdrawn, and quiet each time. She had always been a sparkling and avidly forthcoming conversationalist, so this change was disturbing. We had become good friends, and I missed her affectionate greetings.

Talking with her daughters, they would not acknowledge the obvious. Even at her death, they couldn't accept it. Another troubling factor in dealing with Alzheimer's - never admitting the symptoms' presence, let alone the disease itself. I know this because I found myself not conceding for many years, primarily to myself, however. Not wanting to admit to the obvious is a method of protecting the person suffering from the disease.

At Shirley's funeral, I talked with Chris, Jim's cousin, and she told me she had been visiting with Jim. He was talking about something incoherently that had no basis in reality. Chris said she hadn't realized how far Jim had deteriorated mentally. It had been several years since we had seen them. We talked about Shirley about how she had managed their Italian restaurant for so many years. We talked about the families that came back week after week because of the excellent food. My thought; I think the food was secondary. The reason was that Shirley was such a warm person and made you feel special.

Shirley broke her hip a few years earlier and spent time in the hospital before returning home. She needed extra help for several months. Her daughter, Gina, was managing the restaurant. Shirley died of a heart attack, so ultimately the Alzheimers disease hadn't developed as rapidly. She also had full-time care because the daughters were working and could afford to have someone come in full time. With Shirley diagnosed, another example, and perhaps it confirms my theory of an inherited tendency to Alzheimer's - Jim, his sister, and his mother. Another example, my brother's wife, his mother-in-law, and his daughter all suffered from Alzheimer's disease.

We were living in a house overlooking Puget Sound, and I was recovering emotionally to some extent. Now with the sale of the farm finally completed, we filed a complaint against the Realtor. Included was my narrative of the circumstances and affidavits from the second lawyer and my two sisters. The testimonies depicted the errors throughout the process. I explained the ultimate physical and medical results the agent's behavior caused. My sister Helen added her knowledge, in person, of how my health was affected.

The examining board threw out a section of our complaint because Jim hadn't attended the hearing. But then, what was one more detail added to the debacle that became the sale of our property? At the inquiry with the Real Estate Licensing Board, The decision was, they would put a letter of reprimand in the agent's file. What a silly resolution – who would take the trouble to go to Helena to examine her record?. Ridiculous. A month later, she was running for a position as a trustee for the Flathead Community College. I debated whether I should contact the review board and tell them of her incompetence and lack of ethics. I decided not to and sometimes regretted my decision. But she didn't win, so that helped my resolve.

I'm not sure why we didn't file a complaint against the

original lawyer. We should have; that's obvious. I was troubled and distressed, almost to the point of being hysterical; I probably decided I should put it out of my mind and forget it.

Following the move, I hoped we could let go of the upheaval we had undergone with the property and have a break from anxiety. Up to a point, this was true. With a more structured lifestyle, I found the memory episodes were less stressful. A fixed routine helped Jim to be more at ease and less confused.

In 1995 we sold the house in Mukilteo and moved to Tacoma to be closer to Becki and her family. Because of a conflict in scheduling, Jim had an appointment with a doctor the same day the moving van would arrive. I asked Becki to meet the movers at the house to oversee the unloading because of the appointment. She told me that her father was very agitated when we returned. Jim accused her of wanting us to move so she could take over our finances. She tried to reassure him, explaining that wasn't true, but she thought he probably wasn't convinced. At times he was wildly irrational and couldn't be dissuaded. Ten minutes later, he would have forgotten his accusation, but the hurt inflicted remained.

She understood it was a delusion. Part of the memory problems and frustration he was undergoing and not a personal attack against her. However, it was tough to shrug off such accusations and not feel hurt and bewildered. I told her about his allegation that I hired a man to take over our finances and the farm's operation while still in Montana. One of the more troubling and painful symptoms is the suspicions and suspected ulterior motives of family members. "You don't remember who they are, but you know they are up to no good." It's disheartening and hurtful and hard to put aside even though you know it's part of the disease.

An appointment with a specialist, and he did a series of memory tests to determine the extent of dementia. He reviewed Jim's medical history, checked his past illnesses and current prescriptions (Jim had none). The doctor performed mental status testing to study cognitive skills and a sense of well-being. The doctor's attitude was offensive to me. He was opinionated and arrogant. The doctor talked to me, ignoring Jim sitting beside me. He discussed Jim's condition as if Jim wasn't aware of the surroundings, as if he wasn't in the room. The doctor flat out said it was Alzheimer's. I had already committed my mind to that, having studied what research was available. I was appalled at the doctor's attitude. At the car, as we were leaving, Jim told me he would never go back there. He was aware that day but soon drifted back into confusion. I positively agreed and vowed I would never subject him to such treatment again. When I told Jan about the visit, Jan said he knew the guy from a medical internship, and he did not have a proper manner with people then. Jan was not surprised at the doctor's attitude.

We contacted a different doctor. He did a physical exam and a neurological exam, and a series of mental tests. We discussed other family members who might have been affected by some form of dementia. I informed him about Jim's mother. I explained that she would not see a doctor; therefore, she had not been diagnosed. Observing her symptoms, I suspected Winnie had Alzheimer's. At that time, I was aware Shirley was having health problems. But I learned later that she had symptoms very similar to what Jim was undergoing. It was unsettling to discover that this dreadful, debilitating disease had struck three in my family.

Becki found a group of naturopathic doctors, and we had appointments at their clinic over several months. They offered a plan with vitamins and supplements they said helped in some cases. However, Jim's condition didn't respond, and we discontinued the visits. During these visits, Jim again declared that Becki was trying to take all his money. She was trying to destroy him financially, and he insisted that we had to be careful. This weird idea lasted a month or so. But then he was lucid and responsive and didn't have a memory lapse again for several months.

Later that summer, Jim began having flashbacks, remembering various things but confused about when they happened. Something he hadn't mentioned in years. Bo had died of complications of old age and kidneys shortly after the move to Mukilteo. Jim occasionally looked for her, asking why he couldn't find her. Even though I told him every time he asked, he continued to search. A friend in Montana raised Miniature Schnauzers, and we fell in love with a tiny female and named her Sadie. The arrival of Sadie satisfied his search for Bo. Sadie became one of my helpmates in dealing with the continuing issues of Alzheimer's.

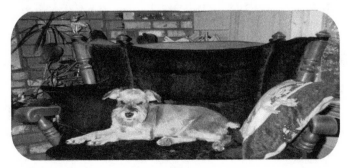

Sadie

Twelve

One of the constant and unsettling problems in dealing with Alzheimer's is the occasional incontinence. Jim wasn't always sure when he had to go to the bathroom. I had to monitor the time, so I could take him after a certain length of time if he seemed agitated. If Jim couldn't find the bathroom, he might go wherever he happened to be. Jim once peed into a paper sack of magazines I planned to deliver to the recycle. I wasn't quick enough to stop him. The magazines didn't make it to recycle, the trash instead.

The doctor prescribed Aricept, a drug that had been somewhat successful in slowing the progression of the disease. The drug had some side effects in the early stages of use. It caused diarrhea, and he couldn't control it. Along with diarrhea, constipation was a recurring problem and triggered a backache we finally discovered was an impacted bowel. From then on, I gave him a teaspoon of Metamucil every day, which took care of constipation. But the alternating bouts of diarrhea and constipation continued to be a problem.

Jim began taking walks around the block with Sadie. I didn't worry about him because Sadie would bring them home. Some days he didn't want to walk and became very agitated if he was outside. Because Jim couldn't remember where he was, the house became a refuge. Jim would only go out if I went with him. As I pulled weeds in the front garden one afternoon, Jim came out and wanted to go for a walk. He said he would take Sadie along, but she pulled back on the leash, sat down, and wouldn't move. That seemed very strange because she always wanted to walk and had been eager to go. Frequently she would bring her leash and sit down in front of him, begging to walk.

I had a fleeting thought that today was different somehow and wondered why.

I brought a lawn chair and suggested he sit for a few minutes, and we could take a ride. He said, "OK," and sat down. I glanced up, and he was gone. I called for him, but there was no answer. I looked up and down the street and called his name again, but he was nowhere in sight. How could he have disappeared so quickly without me noticing? I took the car and drove slowly back and forth through our streets without a sign of him. An hour or so passed, and I decided to go back to the house and call for help. As I opened the door, the phone was ringing. It was a UPS driver several miles away. He said he had found my husband wandering and vague and seemed to be lost. The driver searched Jim's wallet, found his name and telephone number. It was sheer luck, I thought to put the information there. The driver gave me the address and said he would talk to Jim to keep him there and wait for me.

Jim wouldn't leave the house for several days. He seemed to be frightened by any unusual noise. If the television was too loud, he jumped and mumbled. The reaction was different from anything that happened before. I vowed I would watch and observe any other changes and write a note to remember to ask the doctor.

I installed a security system, so if a door or window opened, an alarm would sound. I also decided I had to be entirely sure the system was armed, which proved satisfactory at first. I didn't want any other situations like the UPS episode.

It wasn't long before the next occurrence. Jim slipped out and disappeared within minutes. I hadn't heard the alarm, so he must have figured out how to turn it off and was becoming a perpetual nuisance. Again, I couldn't find him, so I called the police rather than waste time, and a very sympathetic officer came to help. She took his picture and a description and put an alert on the radio. A while later, another police officer called and said he had found him across town, at least ten miles away.

Following my explanation of the situation, the officer suggested I get Jim a cell phone. I explained I had tried that, but he couldn't remember using it, so that idea was useless. I investigated a wrist alarm, but they are audible only 300 yards or so, which wouldn't solve the wandering problem. It was amazing to me that he could disappear and be out of sight so quickly. The reason I mention this; considering the fact, he tended to shuffle and walk at a slow pace.

Several weeks passed without incident, but back to the family room incident. While Jim was napping, I was putting clothes in the washer. When I went back, he was gone. I refuse to believe Jim had turned it off, but the alarm had inadvertently been disarmed. However, I know I didn't turn it off. Anything is possible, I guess. A strange phenomenon of the disease is the ability to dismantle a security system, or in the hotel, the security lock. Sometimes a lucid moment causes consternation, and in our case, locks were often a problem.

Following a search of the house, I looked in the garage, and the pickup was gone. To this day, I don't know how he found the keys. I had hidden them long ago. He wasn't supposed to be driving and hadn't been for at least two years. I called the police again and then went around, hoping to see the pickup but not expecting to. A police alert to locate him was sent by radio. The fear in the pit of my stomach was more intense than ever.

I called Becki, and she and Mike came to the house. We drove through the area and searched for hours. Finally, giving up, we decided to wait to hear from the Highway Patrol. They said they would find him and not to worry. We suggested Mike should try to sleep, and we would wake him if we heard anything. He said he would lie down but probably couldn't fall asleep, but he did.

Jim had been missing for thirteen hours. We were trying not to panic but not having much success. Around 3 a.m., the telephone rang. It was a highway patrolman calling from Wenatchee, off Interstate 90. He told me he recognized the pickup and license from the APB and pulled Jim over. I said to the officer, "My husband wasn't supposed to be driving. I think he was going back to Montana." The officer laughed. "He was doing a pretty good job for somebody who wasn't supposed to be driving. He was going the speed limit and definitely knew where he was headed. He didn't offer any resistance. But I think he's very tired." The patrolman said he would take my husband to a motel and instruct the clerk to call him if Jim should decide to leave before we could get there. He locked the pickup and would leave the key with the motel clerk.

We left immediately and reached the motel about 11:30 in the morning. We paid and thanked the clerk, collected Jim and a pizza he had bought somewhere during his trip. We ate breakfast nearby before leaving for home. Becki drove the pickup, and I followed her in my car. Jim didn't remember anything about what happened. He kept patting my shoulder and remarking every three or four minutes that it was a beautiful day for a drive. I made a mental note to find a better place to hide the key. I also had to double-check the security system to be sure it was still armed. I was beginning to think Jim might

121

have figured out how to turn it off during one of his lucid moments.

One day I asked him to wait in the car for a few minutes while I ran into the grocery for several items. When I went to the check-out, Jim came up with our little dog Sadie in a cart. I asked the checker why she hadn't told him to leave, and she said he wasn't causing a problem, and she had no objection to him with the dog in the cart. She was compassionate and caring, even knowing dogs weren't supposed to be in the store. Such a sweet lady. I couldn't leave Jim in the car for more than a few minutes because he became agitated, and I was concerned he might decide to leave.

It was a year or so before we had another severe episode. I was fixing lunch when I heard the door chime and went to see where Jim was. He must have unlocked the door because it was open, and he was gone, and the pickup was gone. How in the world was my first thought? I looked up and down the street, no pickup in sight. I immediately called the police to alert them again. They didn't locate him but would keep searching. As the hours passed, I fretted and paced, trying to stay calm. I was nearing total panic. Beck and her husband were equally concerned. Mike was agitated that his Grampa was missing again.

It's gut-wrenching, wondering where he is and what might be happening. You imagine all sorts of terrible outcomes. Because you know how confusing everything is to him, you think of all the possibilities of something horrible. The waiting to hear something – good or bad – is almost unbearable. But over the years, you have accustomed yourself, I guess, to expect the unexpected. There is the fear in the pit of your stomach that never completely goes away. There is always the feeling that something dreadful will happen, and try as you might; you can't keep it buried.

A day and a half later, I received a telephone call from the Sheriff in Eugene, Oregon. The Sheriff told me they had my husband at the station. A grocery store clerk noticed a man walking back and forth in front of the store. "He seemed to be in distress, so I asked him, what's the matter? He was disoriented and couldn't tell me his name or where he lived. I called the Sheriff to find out what to do." The Sheriff took Jim to the station, and they found our phone number in his wallet. The Sheriff arranged for Jim to stay at a senior center, and the lady there said she would feed him and take care of him until someone could come.

I called Jan, and he flew to Eugene. My son said the lady at the shelter was amiable, and he tried to pay her, but she resisted vehemently, saying she was glad to help. Jan drove the pickup back to our home. They were both worn out. I helped Jim with a shower and fixed breakfast, and they slept for hours. I am so grateful when I think about what could have happened without those thoughtful people and how they helped us through a difficult situation.

I wrote to the store, the Sheriff, and the Senior Center to thank them for caring. Sometimes the burden was heavy, and it took an effort to remind myself that I wasn't in this alone. But it was discouraging to see a once vibrant, active man retreat into the fogginess that had become his life.

The disease was progressing steadily. There were no longer extended periods when Jim was his old self. Only rarely did he remember Becki or Mike, although they were at our house often. Because Jim saw me every day and knew me but didn't always remember my name. Nights he became restless and didn't sleep more than an hour at a time. I had to be aware, so I guess I slept with one eye open, as that weird saying goes.

Consequently, I wasn't getting much sleep. Days had become nights, and nights had become days. Interrupted sleep is defined as moonlighting and is a symptom of Alzheimer's. Jim would often move to the sofa and sleep a few hours, whether day or night. The wandering during the night is called sundowning. It is a disruption, whatever it is named. In our battle with Alzheimer's, sundowning was a continuing problem.

In the afternoon, he watched Jeopardy, one television show he enjoyed. It was odd that only one program caught his attention. Experts speculate that people with Alzheimer's might see television differently. Perhaps they only see images, and that may be why they lose the ability to recognize people. Most days, Jim had no concept of time or where he was. He needed help with daily activities such as dressing or showering. However, all through the ordeal, he could feed himself. Alzheimers patients sometimes lose that ability. Chocolate chip cookies were a special favorite. But those particular cookies were a favorite from when he was a little boy. My daughter and her husband brought a cookie back from a trip. It was the size of a dinner plate, and Jim couldn't have been more pleased. We cut it into smaller pieces so he could enjoy it for days.

As the disease progressed, he did not recognize people and occasionally would ask me, "Who are you?" He was irritable when he was aware of his surroundings, which happened very seldom now. Irritability is another sign of Alzheimer's, and doctors suspect the culprit might be a vitamin deficiency. I had noticed this in Jim's mother. If I could convince her to take her vitamins, she was more alert that day.

Something that seemed to be unusual is the fact that Jim wanted ice cream all the time. Not remembering, he had finished a bowlful, and a few minutes later, he wanted another. I asked the doctor, and he said to give it to him. It won't hurt; it'll help keep him calm. Becki was sitting with him one day so that I could run an errand. She said he asked if she wanted ice cream at least twenty times over the two hours she stayed.

I discussed some ideas with Jan and Minde. One concern was guns. Over the years, Jim had collected a few rifles and handguns. I had hidden the bullets. But Minde said if Jim went outside waving a pistol, a police officer might use force, not knowing but assuming the gun was loaded. An accident of this kind was unthinkable but a possibility. Minde is a retired detective, and I listened to her concerns, which mirrored what I thought. Jan took all the guns when they went back to their home. That worry was gone. Occasionally, if something upset him, he said he had a pool cue, and it was a good weapon if he needed one. It was not clear, of course, why he might need it. Furthermore, we did not have a pool cue.

Thirteen

I was reaching the point of total exhaustion. I needed some respite and time to attend to errands. I investigated our health insurance policy, and the company claimed we weren't covered. The agent who had sold the plan said that was not true. She read the particular clause that described home health. After weeks of telephone calls and letters and arguing, they finally concluded the policy did cover our situation. They settled to have a helper come in for two hours three times a week. Having those few hours were a godsend. I could relax for a time, even if only to run to the drugstore or grocery.

One young woman was accommodating and helpful. She was so attentive to Jim and could anticipate his needs. One day, she came with her husband and four-year-old son and said they wanted to take Jim for a drive and stop for ice cream. She was thoughtful and helped with many chores, dusting, vacuuming, and putting groceries in the cupboards. Reading to Jim, he was calm, although I'm not sure he understood what she read. With Jim's increasing frustration and anxiety. When it became too difficult, even with relief, I had to investigate options. When I finally decided to take him to the care facility, she asked if she could stop by and visit him. Of course, she could. She was a gem.

My sister, Helen, came to visit from California, and we toured several nursing homes and rest homes. Some were awful. They had a foul smell and were more like a tomb than a natural home. We found Pioneer Place, a nursing home with an Alzheimer's wing. It was new and comfortable. We talked with the staff, and they appeared to be caring and professional.

I mentioned that Jim loved ice cream, and the attendant said they could have it any time they wanted, and they always had cookies in the afternoon.

The manager from Pioneer Place came to the house to meet Jim and discuss the situation. She asked probing questions while observing him. He was in his favorite chair, alternating between watching Jeopardy and dozing off. She inquired if he was violent or had ever been. He had never exhibited any signs of violence, except verbally.

Or an occasion when he thought someone had been stealing from him. At those times, he said he should use a pool cue to get his stuff back. We did not have a pool cue. In a few minutes, he had forgotten he was angry and drifted back into the fuzziness of his mind. I explained Jim's flashes of anger if he commented, and someone disagreed, but they happened very rarely now. We had discussed with Mike not to argue with his grampa but agree even if it was a ridiculous statement or if he repeated the same sentence numerous times. It usually helped.

In July, we arranged a week's trial to see if the place was a fit. During that week, I went to Montana with Becki to visit friends, my niece, and three older sisters. When we returned, the Manager told me Jim had been just fine, no problems. They would be glad to have him as a resident. She gave me a list of what he would need, and we moved him into his room. A young woman, a nurse, said she would look out for him. We provided a television so he could watch jeopardy. They mentioned I should take his wristwatch with me because another resident would take it. She said she was tired of having to hunt for possessions that were mislaid or borrowed. She said she didn't like to say stolen because they probably did not realize something belonged to that particular person.

.Years earlier, we had the foresight to secure a long-term-care insurance policy. I applied for coverage of the cost of Pioneer Place. The insurance company denied the claim saying the content didn't apply to the facility. Their assertion that the Pioneer Place Statement of Intent filed with the State Licensing Board did not cover the care offered. There was a conflict because the mission statement was in a different category in their operating license. The Insurance company claimed the policy did not cover custodial care, which Jim needed; assistance with dressing, showering, eating, walking, and other daily activities.

Arguing against such nonsense, I spent countless hours on the telephone and writing letters. I contacted everyone I could think of for help, legislators, newspapers, an attorney, and the policy's agent. The pressure from her is what made the insurance company decide to change the decision. After a month and a half, it was adjusted to our benefit by the claims official. I deeply resent the hours it took away. The time that should have been spent with Jim those last months when he needed me. I found the insurance companies to be an obstacle and suggest a careful review of the actual coverage.

The staff at Pioneer Place welcomed him with hugs and helped him adjust by serving him ice cream and cookies. One young nurse took a particular liking to him. She said he reminded her of her grandfather. She helped with Jim's transition from home to new surroundings, so the change wouldn't be scary for him. They told me later; the night staff groused about him when he wandered and peed in the corner instead of visiting the bathroom. I explained he probably couldn't find it or didn't remember where to go. The janitors understood, of course, because they were familiar with such accidents.

One day a tiny lady came running down the hallway, waving her arms. She didn't have a stitch of clothes on. The nurse told me she was their resident nudist. She took her clothes off all the time, and they had to catch her and put them back on, and she would take them off again as soon as they left her.

I went every Tuesday, Thursday, and Sunday to visit. One day I picked Jim up at 10 a.m. for a dental appointment. Becki accompanied me, and we planned to go to lunch and stop for ice cream. The dentist took less than an hour, and we enjoyed a pleasant afternoon. Arriving back at Pioneer Place, Jim didn't want to get out of the car. He realized we were not at our house. We went in with him, thinking that he might be calmer after we stayed a while. His favorite nurse stopped and asked about his trip to town and distracted him. We didn't want to go if he continued to plead with us not to leave him. We sat with him and a half-hour or so, and later, he began to listen to music on television. He didn't notice when we said goodbye and left.

At the end of the month, there was a birthday celebration for everyone with a birthday. The residents didn't remember whose birthday or what holiday they were celebrating. The staff arranged a visiting music program every month and spent time with each person to not feel neglected or overlooked. I took Sadie with me on every visit, and she went from person to person to be petted and cooed over. She seemed to know which person needed extra time and would sit on a lap and snuggle.

One of the music visits was a Hawaiian program. The

dancers passed out leis to the residents, and one lady put her's on Sadie, and everyone clapped. They were delighted that day and sang along with the music. A staff member took a picture of Sadie and put it on the bulletin board alongside a picture of the lady giving Sadie the lei.

On one occasion, a man picked Sadie up, insisting she was his dog. He wouldn't let go of her, and I was worried he would squeeze her in his determination. He wasn't willing to put her down. One of the staff coaxed him into sitting down and holding her on his lap. She talked him into releasing Sadie by telling him she was tired and needed to rest for a while. He agreed, and she solved the problem without mishap to little Sadie. The nurse said that his dog had died. His son said they couldn't let him have another dog because he was not responsible enough. We felt such sympathy for him.

In September, Jan and Minde drove from Spokane, and we spent a Sunday with Jim at Pioneer Place. We took him seedless grapes (his favorite snack). He sat with us but appeared listless and vague. I'm not sure he remembered them, even though I reminded him. We chatted, mainly with each other. Jim smiled now and then, and Jan commented that maybe he was tired. We stayed a few hours, and the kids hugged him as we left. I told him I would be back on Tuesday, and he responded with a smile and patted my shoulder.

On Tuesday, Jim was very vague, much more than usual. Sadie sat on his lap, and he stroked her absentmindedly. He wasn't anxious or agitated. On the Thursday visit, Jim was lying in bed. The nurse said he had been in bed all day and having trouble breathing. I asked if the doctor had seen him, and she said yes, but he didn't seem concerned. I asked Jim if he wanted to sit up, and he said, "yes." The nurse helped him dress. I turned on his television, and we sat for a few hours. He kept patting my shoulder and seemed contented, but his breathing was ragged. He repeated over and over how glad he was to see me, and this was unusual. Because some days he didn't speak at all. He alternated between patting my shoulder and patting Sadie lying on his lap. He was very lethargic, and I asked the nurse to check again with the doctor, and she said she would.

He wasn't upset when I mentioned I had to take Sadie home and feed her, and I would be back on Sunday. Jim mumbled something I couldn't understand, and hugging him, I left. I was exhausted and went to bed early. I was awakened at eleven by the telephone ringing. It was the nurse from Pioneer Place. She said Jim had pneumonia, and they were taking him to the hospital. She said I should wait until morning and try not to worry. I couldn't sleep but dozed fitfully, tossing and turning. I thought this is crazy, and I have to do something. After a cup of coffee and feeding Sadie, I drove to the hospital.

I arrived at the Tacoma Hospital early Friday morning. Approaching the nurse's station, I inquired about where to find my husband. He wasn't there, and there was no record but a notation that they didn't have a bed. I explained about the midnight arrival from Pioneer Place, and the nurse on duty said she would call other hospitals. I think she was concerned about me because she said, "We'll find him, don't you worry."

Two other hospitals also had no beds, but the third hospital told us he was brought there by ambulance and had been there for a half-hour. But they didn't have a bed available. He was transferred back to the ambulance and taken to St Clair's about

30 miles south. I drove to the hospital, and he was in the acute care section. When I finally found him, the nurse told me he had been asking for me for hours. Upon my arrival, he calmed down and quit fighting the oxygen and IV line. I asked the doctor how Jim was doing and when or if he could go home, and the doctor said, "No, he's too sick."

I sat beside the bed, holding his hand, and he relaxed somewhat. I sat with him for several hours until I had to go home to feed Sadie and take her out briefly. I called the children to tell them their dad was in the hospital. Jan spoke to the doctor on duty, and after talking to him, Jan phoned Becki and Pat to explain the situation with their father.

I went to the hospital early Saturday morning. The doctor said Jim's condition had worsened and that everyone should come immediately. The pneumonia was deadly, and the antibiotics did not touch it. It was only a matter of time. They could make him comfortable and help with his breathing. The doctor commented on how strong Jim's heartbeat was, considering he had smoked for over 50 years and breathed diesel smoke from 43 years on the railroad. Emphysema had taken a toll on his lungs.

The family living in the area gathered. Because only two people were allowed at a time, we took turns in the room. Pat was on his way from Wisconsin but would not arrive until after eight. Jan and Minde were driving from Spokane. We were still taking turns sitting with Jim between the nurses, clearing his lungs, and checking his breathing. At one o'clock, the doctor said we should all go in. It was time. Becki wanted him to know we were there. She asked the doctor if her Dad could hear us. The doctor said he thought Jim could if we wanted to say "goodbye."

Jim died at two-thirty the afternoon of September 22nd, 2001. Even with the oxygen, he had congestion and labored breathing. My husband quietly slipped away while I held his hand. Jan and Minde came in the door a few minutes after he died. They were not on time to say goodbye, and Pat had not arrived.

Jim's long twilight struggle was over. Losing him was unbearably painful, but it was the end of his excruciating ordeal. It was many years earlier that we really lost him. His body was there, but he was not the husband and father we loved. Jim's frustration, the wasting away, memory deterioration, anxiety, and dependency was heartbreaking to watch. He was a proud man, and with his zest for living, he would have hated what his life had become.

We held a memorial in Whitefish. The priest from the Episcopal Church where Jim was baptized presided. Comments included his time in the Navy. Two of his friends from the railroad each gave a eulogy. His hunting buddy, John, remarked about Jim often saying something was pusillanimous. John said he didn't know what that meant, but it always fit whatever happened when Jim said it. People I had never seen before attended and offered sympathy. Jan said he had a lengthy visit with the priest. They talked about Jan growing up in Whitefish and our participation in the church. We reminisced with some of the people Jim had known for a lifetime. His kindness and generosity had touched the hearts of numerous friends and acquaintances. My three oldest sisters helped soothe the ache in our hearts. They had each lost a husband, and Evelyn had suffered the loss of a son as well. He died of cancer when he was seventeen. She said not a day went by that she didn't think of him.

We scattered Jim's ashes at his favorite fishing spot on the North Fork of the Flathead River. A marble stone at the gravesite of his Father and Mother signifies Jim's service to the country he loved. Shirley added a stone marker for Winnifred. They are now together.

I miss him, his gentleness, his love of books, crossword puzzles, and a game of solitaire he invented. I miss the enjoyable conversation and the life we had. I miss the travel we never had--planned for after retirement. Sometimes a song or a joke will trigger the thought, "Jim would certainly have liked that," and I struggle against tears. We had fifty-one years together, but I especially miss the time stolen from us.

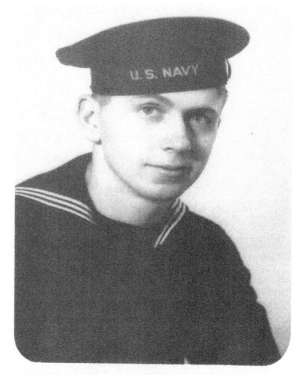

Jim – Navy – South Pacific

Fourteen

Many families are coping with this debilitating disease. I include four stories of someone touched by Alzheimer's. I think their suffering should be acknowledged and remembered.

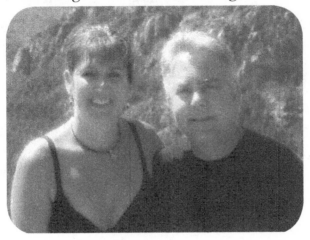

Kim and Pat

Carlotta

My son Pat's wife also had a personal experience with the disease. Her mother, Carlotta, struggled for years, but some of the situations and conditions differed from my experiences. Carlotta's husband was the primary caregiver in her case. Carlotta paced back and forth in the house. Carlotta wandered away twice. When I first met Carlotta, she was lucid and aware. Although ironing a tablecloth, she continued in the same spot until Kim mentioned it. At that point, Carlotta said, "I'm done, put the iron away. "

She folded and unfolded towels incessantly. I've wondered if the repetitive action helps control the frustration. But, this is just my thought, no scientific basis.

Carlotta belonged to a painting class, and her oils were colorful and very lovely. Even as the disease progressed, she continued to spend time with her art, but it deteriorated in quality. The paintings began to look more like a third-grader, and it bothered her terribly. Finally, she didn't remember how to mix colors. She had always been precise. It was becoming more and more frustrating, and she quit painting altogether.

Carlotta became very frightened if left alone for any length of time. In the last year of her life, she began having fainting episodes and sometimes fell. Her husband called 911. Carlotta spent a couple of visits to the hospital until the doctor decided it resulted from Alzheimer's and deteriorating brain activity. Toward the end of her life, she couldn't speak words, she could only mumble, and her speech was garbled and couldn't be understood.

Both of Carlotta's parents had Alzheimer's. She worried about herself and looked for signs of it happening. But Carlotta wouldn't talk about it, and she ignored it. Carlotta's mother had flashes of anger, similar to Jim's, but her father didn't experience that. We discussed the anger issue. The grandkids were told that the rage wasn't directed toward them but inward, indicating something was wrong. I explained that to my grandson about not arguing with his Grampa.

Carlotta's husband was her caregiver for all five to seven years as the disease progressed. He took her to the senior center for an afternoon for a while but finally resorted to outside help. During Carlotta's last year, a home-care person came in for six hours every day except Sunday. However, eventually, the service went seven days a week.

Carlotta was injured in an automobile accident, crashing her head. After suffering a severe brain injury, there is convincing evidence that Carlotta's accident was probably the beginning of the symptoms. In Carlotta's case, the Alzheimers progressed over approximately ten years. Whereas, in my husband's case, it was closer to twenty years. Quite often, in the latter stages of the illness, bodily functions stop. Her body quit working, and her kidneys shut down. The muscles in her bowels didn't work anymore. Everything was closing down and no longer functioning. The doctors could have done surgery to help. The family decided an operation would be too drastic and would not benefit the underlying problem of Alzheimer's. Carlotta was at home when she died with her family around her. She was only sixty-nine.

Carlotta had a brain injury. In my husband's case, Jim had two severe blows to the head, with a period of unconsciousness in the train accident injury.

Mary

My brother's wife, Mary, contracted Alzheimer's. Mel had died years earlier, so luckily, he did not have to cope with his wife's deterioration. Their daughter told me it started with forgetting. Mary didn't remember what day it was and couldn't remember where she was. She didn't wander away. However, Thelma became concerned about leaving her mother alone while at work. Her daughter said Mary was overly friendly. If someone walked by, Mary would go out and ask them to come in for coffee. She didn't know the passersby, but in her dementia, they had to be someone she knew if they were by her house.

Mary, at that point, didn't recognize people but thought she should because they were there. It was strange to come into the house, and people would be sitting in the kitchen. They looked bewildered, wondering what was going on, and she would explain about the Alzheimers. Most of the time, people understood and were sympathetic.

Mary thought that Virgilio, our Dad, was Mel's Dad but not ours. She couldn't relate that we were Mel's sisters. I hadn't seen her for a few years until my sister Vera's funeral. Mary didn't know me, but she was friendly. While talking with us, she rambled, making no sense. It didn't bother me because we were familiar with the symptoms. We listened and nodded occasionally.

Mary had other health problems. When admitted to the hospital, she needed a catheter. However, she didn't understand and was very upset. Mary wanted to get out of bed and go to the bathroom. She couldn't comprehend what was happening. The Doctor suggested that Mary should be in a nursing home to have the care she needed. Following the doctor's advice, they complied. She adjusted reasonably well, but she wrote all the time. Nothing that made sense, and she deteriorated to a child level. But she kept writing and writing. After a while, she would not talk, not even mumble. Mary suffered a stroke, and the facility called another daughter. However, it took twenty minutes to arrive, and Mary succumbed to a second stroke. Mary's daughter was not in time to say goodbye to her mother. Mary lived at the long-term-care facility for four years. She was eighty-four when she died. Two workers from the Care Center attended the funeral. They said they were fond of Mary because she was a sweet person.

Jum & Muz

Nellie

Mary's mother, Nellie Jarrett, also contracted Alzheimer's. She was very aware, off and on, for a long time. I didn't know Nellie well because I only saw her occasionally. I do remember her little dog. Nellie told me that whenever they went for groceries, they always brought a cabbage for the dog. She loved it and ate the whole head in one sitting.

Mary, Melvin, and four children lived with Nellie on a property that her great-grandfather had homesteaded. Nellie quit-claimed the property to Mary before she deteriorated and wouldn't know what was happening. Their daughter told me her grandmother wanted the homestead taken care of because she knew something was wrong. Nellie was upset at her condition and suffered anxiety and frustration.

She wanted to leave the property to her daughter, Mary. But, before Nellie's planned move into a nursing home or to receiving Medicaid, state law determined it must be seven years before a transfer. Oddly enough, it was seven years and one month before Nellie's admittance, and she was a resident in the nursing home for only a year. She became very debilitated and curled up in a fetal position. Toward the end of her life, Nellie was fragile. She was also 84 when she died.

Carol

Carol is a daughter of Mary and a granddaughter of Nellie, and a sister to Jewel and Thelma. Carol is the third member of the family to develop Alzheimer's. It began with eight years of forgetfulness and memory loss. Thelma became concerned, but the first doctor they talked with didn't believe the family when they explained Carol's situation. Another doctor in September of 2019 diagnosed her with probable Parkinson's and Alzheimer's. He performed several tests. He followed an MRI with a spinal tap to check for pressure on the brain, and the tap came up negative. When Carol could not be left alone, and Thelma had to work, the family decided to follow the doctor's advice. They looked for a place where she would be safe and receive the help she needed.

In November of 2019, they were fortunate to admit Carol to the Benefis Senior Services Memory Care Home in Great Falls, Montana. Jewel's husband, a minister, had been conducting a monthly service. He also held weekly prayer groups. For over eight years, he was always available if needed. The staff welcomed Caro,l, and Jewel commented on the warm response to her as well.

Jewel visits every few days, but Carol does not recognize her. Carol won't walk and will not get out of bed. The staff devised a sling to bring her to a wheelchair. She will eat once they have her situated in the dining room. Carol has enjoyed the sling. Jewel said the staff told her that Carol yells, "Whoopee." They have to keep her door closed because she takes her clothes off. The doctor mentioned that it is a sign of reverting to childhood. Carol is 78 years old, and Jewel thinks she seems happy. She no longer recognizes anyone and is in a wheelchair full-time. She was always a happy person. When I speak with Jewel on the phone, I hear the pain in her voice, and I understand it. I have mentioned to the sisters that I will support them and offered help if they need it.

A Footnote

I have thought to myself and questioned something; Jim's mother was 84, Mary was 84, and her mother Nellie was 84 when they died. Is there a pattern here? Jim might have lived to be that age if he had not succumbed to pneumonia. He was 75 when he died, but his heartbeat was still strong, and he had not yet suffered the shutting down of bodily functions. Of course, I can only speculate about this. Alzheimer's can strike at any age and develop over a short amount of time or progress over many years.

Loving Remembrance

James Stuart Connelly, Jr. Winnifred Horton Connelly

Shirley Connelly Orlando   Carlotta Inorio Matta

Mary Jarrett Ambrogini   Nellie Jarrett

Hugh

Hugh was Jim's friend since first grade and a considerable part of our lives. I include Hugh's story because of their long friendship. I Forget' is dedicated to (Jum) and his battle with Alzheimer's.

Hugh Roberts was born in 1921 and grew up in Whitefish, Montana. The railroad tracks divided the town side and the lake side in the small town. Hugh was a leader of the lakeside boys. Although he was five years older, he looked out for them. My husband Jim was one of the boys, with Rex, Larry, and Harold. They lived within a few blocks of each other and stayed friends over the next fifty years.

There was a friendly feud between the kids from town and Lakeside. They made slingshots out of strips from old rubber inner-tubes and shot rocks at each other. The town kids had to cross the viaduct to Whitefish Lake to swim. That instigated some of the rivalries between the town kids and the lakeside kids. It is incredible to me that no one was injured or killed, but the times were simple. I guess kids had tremendous freedom, and parents were more lenient, that's for sure.

In 1938 the school in the lakeside of the town burned to the ground. Officials of the Great Northern Railroad provided a railroad car for the students while construction was underway to rebuild the school. The railroad was the primary industry. Italians and a few Japanese helped build the railroad when it came to Whitefish in 1904. However, logging was also predominant at that time. Logs floated downriver were loaded and transported on freight cars. Children in the lakeside of Whitefish attended the makeshift school, Jim and Hugh among them.

Following graduation from the University with an engineering degree, Hugh joined the Army. The government was conducting a project in Oak Ridge, Tennessee. The government delegation asked members of Hugh's unit if anyone was an engineer. A few were chosen, including Hugh, and were involved in the program for eighteen months. It was very hush-hush. They were gathering information to build the atomic bomb. However, Hugh told us he didn't know what they were working on until much later.

The government provided housing, but the engineers were not allowed to leave the complex. Divided into groups, they were kept separate and did not know how other engineers were involved. The men found out what the project entailed when the atomic bombs were deployed and dropped on Japan. He said a few of them suspected but did not talk about it. He was not aware at the time. It was all top secret, of course. He wonders, and it is still a mystery to him. How was the Manhattan Project kept a secret before being launched?

The war ended, and Hugh hired on with GE. He traveled the east coast setting up steam turbines and significant projects. Each of the various jobs would last a month or a couple of months. He said he was never in one place long enough to make close friends. Consequently, after several years he quit and returned to Whitefish. He went to work as a Fireman on the Great Northern Railroad. He was promoted to Locomotive Engineer, just as Jim was.

At that time, Hugh also had the responsibility of helping his mother. She suffered from MS and gradually deteriorated-- from using crutches to a wheelchair. His father had died, and his mother had remarried and was again a widow. He commented one time that their house was two shacks put together and was not worth much. That happened throughout the town as it changed and progressed.

It was after he moved back to Whitefish that I met him. Hugh lived across the street from my husband Jim while growing up. They stayed best friends and kept in touch through college and service during World War II. Jim and I were married, had bought a house, and settled in Whitefish. I had heard the Whitefish stories about the kids in the neighborhood. When Hugh returned, they renewed their friendship. Subsequently, he became an extended part of our family and is godfather to our three kids, Jan, Becki, and Pat.

A friend of Hugh's from his days at GE was a frequent visitor in Whitefish. We met Mabel and grew to love her too. She was an exceptional person, and she made Hugh happy. While visiting, Mabel became fast friends with Jim's mother, Winnifred. When Winnie began having health problems, we bought a house trailer and moved it to our farm. She did not want to live with us, but we wanted her close. We could help if necessary.

Our dog, Bo, decided to guard Winnie as part of her job. Bo snarled at everyone except Jim and myself. Bo adopted Winnie as her particular person. It was a strange friendship, but it worked for both of them. I marveled at their closeness, the dog who hated everybody and the cranky older woman who complained about everything except the dog.

Over the years, we had countless cats and dogs. One particular cat was a yellow tom. He had peculiar habits, such as fighting squirrels almost every day. His ears were lopsided, and one eye drooped. He also marked his territory and was a total pain in that respect.

One day Hugh was sitting on the step, Jan was beside him, and I was standing below. We were discussing something about a planned fishing trip. The cat went up behind them on the step and proceeded to pee on Hugh's back. Hugh hollered, and the cat jumped down and ran. "What the hell," Hugh said. "Why would he do that?" We were all equally astounded as to why. The cat did not do anything like that again but continued his other weird habits. The yellow cat was the same one who went with us when we cut a Christmas tree. In some respects, he acted more like a dog rather than a cat. He disappeared one day, and Jim said he probably attacked a moose and was still out there somewhere.

Jim and Hugh enjoyed fishing along with Jay (Jim's father). We included Hugh in Thanksgiving and Christmas celebrations. The kids loved him. He tutored them in math, and they had long conversations about life, coping with problems, and schoolwork. He attended recitals and functions with us. He taught the kids to ice skate and to learn to drive. One summer, they painted his house, and my sister Babe and I painted his garage. Our family Sunday dinners always included Hugh.

On a trip back to Montana, after moving to Washington State, we left Sadie overnight with Hugh. The next day he told us she sat at the window and barked all night. One of his neighbors called to complain. Hugh was tired from lack of sleep. However, Sadie slept the entire day. She was exhausted. I mentioned that we would not leave her again. Hugh was a good sport and said she was homesick for us, and he understood.

Hugh told me one time he was pheasant hunting with Jay, and they went south toward Polson. They climbed over a fence, and the whole area was marshy and wet. As they walked through, they shot their quota and went on toward the road. As they climbed the fence on the opposite side, they noticed a sign. They were in a protected game preserve. The warning on the other barrier had collapsed; at least, it was no longer there. They were unnerved and panicked as to what they should do about the illegal birds. After a lengthy discussion, they thought it might be best to go home and forget about it. He said he still feels guilt about the incident.

When Hugh bought a pickup truck, Jan convinced him to choose several options he probably wouldn't have considered otherwise. The same applied when he bought a car. Hugh was always willing to let the kids state their opinions. A quirk we thought they sometimes carried too far, but if Hugh disagreed, he undoubtedly told them outright.

Hugh liked working with wood, and he built bookcases, dressers, and a gun cabinet. He helped add an addition to our little log house and created the kitchen cabinets of solid birch. They are beautiful as well as functional. Also, he helped me design the plan with cabinets and cubbies to finish the loft.

He taught the boys to shoot at the local rifle range. Pat competed in meets across the Northwest, winning trophies and ribbons. I remember especially one rifle meet in Great Falls during a horrific storm. The wind was so strong while crossing the street, Jim held one of my hands and Hugh the other to keep me from being blown away.

That year a series of storms piled snow to the rooftops, and the wind was especially damaging. The high winds during one storm blew several freight cars off the tracks along the Highline. The Traveling Engineer was slammed against a freight car by the force of the wind. He had just commented that there wasn't a need to worry about the storm. It's a crock, and I don't believe the warnings. "I guess I was wrong about that," was all he said while trying to stand against the wind. In a way, it was funny, but he listened after that when the crew told him something to avoid or what might happen.

Hugh never married and had no children of his own, so our kids and our family became his family. On fishing trips, Hugh and Jim included the kids and the cocker, Rusty. Hugh laughingly told me he always carried the dog across the river. Jim said he finally realized the reason Hugh always offered to lug Rusty was the extra weight. It kept him from being knocked around by the current. The dog story became a running joke, and we still laugh about it if the subject comes up about the North Fork of the Flathead River. Jan and Hugh were incredibly close because they became fast friends before Becki and Pat were born.

Hugh enjoyed the outdoors and liked to cut firewood. Every summer, he took a load to various people. He and Jim sometimes combined their efforts. Jan always wanted to be included, although both boys went multiple times. We had a wood heater and had to stock up enough to last through the winter.

Hugh took his dog, Stick, with him to cut firewood. But on one trip, Stick disappeared. He called and searched but couldn't find him. He went back several times, called and whistled, but the dog didn't respond. Hugh said he didn't want another dog after that experience.

The dog was committed to Hugh, although initially, he belonged to twin boys who lived across the street. Stick moved to Hugh's house, and the boys didn't care. Stick was exceedingly possessive. When Hugh fell and hurt his back and called 911, the dog wouldn't let the paramedics in to help. Finally, one of the guys went to the back door and yelled. The dog charged the door; the paramedics scrambled and were able to take Hugh to the ambulance. We checked the house later to let Stick outside. Hugh went back home the next day, but he had a sore back for several weeks.

Becki was very reticent about people the first year after she was born. It was funny because Hugh wanted to hold her. She always had to sit facing out because if she looked at him, she would cry. I think it hurt Hugh's feelings, but he would never say so. I explained that Becki did that with everybody but eventually quit. We attended meetings when Jan was in Boy Scouts. Pat always wanted to sit on Hugh's lap. Pat had to have his favorite blanket, and if it was accidentally left home, he threw a fit and cried. Hugh would console him. Later, when Pat joined Cub Scouts, Hugh continued to attend events with us. He was fantastic with the kids. Christmas was a favorite for him. Hugh had the kids list things they wanted. I mentioned he was spoiling them, but he said it was his choice.

After the kids moved away, Hugh and Jim continued to enjoy doing things they loved. I remember one particular fishing trip. I dropped the two of them off at a creek toward the Canadian border. I spent the afternoon with my sisters at Fortine, and the guys planned to fish until 4 o'clock.

I arrived a little after four to find them walking along the road, and their jeans and boots were solid with slimy mud. Laughing hilariously, Hugh explained what happened. Jim slipped on the muddy bank and slid into the water. When Hugh tried to pull him out, he slid down the bank, couldn't stop, and ended up in the mud too. I debated whether I should allow them into the car. I threatened to leave them, and we had a good laugh at the ridiculous situation. I put their jackets on the back seat for them to sit on. But I had to clean the car after we arrived home. By the way, they didn't catch any fish.

Several years ago, Hugh moved to a retirement home. It's an enjoyable place. He said he was tired of doing the cooking, and the facility offered three squares a day. Hugh convinced the management to purchase a billiard table. He recruited some of the residents to play poker, although most chose to work on jigsaw puzzles. There was always a card table on the landing with an ongoing puzzle.

Hugh continued long walks almost every day. He drove back to his house three or four times a week, just to sit and ponder. Although, sometimes cleaning one of the guns in his collection and fixing a bowl of soup. He failed his eye exam to renew his driver's license. He was no longer able to drive himself to the house. His independence was diminished and was upsetting and disappointing. Hugh recruited a friend to take him a few times a week.

As the years passed, Hugh became a friend of the children of our children. They learned to shoot with him and were taught to fish as well. Jim and Hugh's closeness and life-long friendship continued through the children, although Jim is no longer with us.

Hugh just passed his 94th birthday and is having health issues. We spent four days with him in January of 2016. He is struggling with a lung condition, a collapse, and fluid build-up. While working on the Railroad, the doctors speculate,

Hugh spent time in Libby, where crews loaded Zonolite onto freight cars for shipment. Dust from the manufacturing was continually blowing back onto the train crew and caused breathing hazards.

The company closed the plant. But meanwhile, people living there and others working there continue to suffer. Research shows it can take many years for the dust to cause lung conditions and other health difficulties. It was following a lawsuit that the plant closed. But company officials have been allowed to get away without being held accountable.

Hugh said he had a long life and is not worried about what his future might hold. He doesn't want us to plan a service, and we have agreed to abide by his wishes. We have enjoyed his friendship over the last 70 years. We will miss him, but we have good memories. When we sat with him over those four days, he was tired but talkative. One of us would ask a question, and we listened to his recollections. We took lots of pictures. He is feeling better, and I hope he continues to improve. We don't want to lose him just yet.

Hugh reminisced about a week the six of us spent in Yellowstone Park in the mid-sixties during our visit. He commented that he has fond memories, and that was the best vacation we had together. We marveled at Old Faithful and the other geysers, the Paint Pots, and the Mineral Hot Springs. We counted over a hundred bears and saw bison, elk, and other wildlife that inhabit the park.

Leaving the park, we spent time at the Lewis and Clark Caverns, Nevada City, and Virginia City. Pat wondered about the two-story outhouse, did stuff from the top-level fall on people on the lower level. A strange thought, I think, for a kid. Becki was primarily interested in seeing the club foot of a notorious outlaw. Jan wanted to see the silver dollar collection in the counter of a combination bar restaurant. Looking back, I agree with Hugh. Everyone said they feel the same. It was the best vacation ever. With the deterioration of Hugh's health, when the time comes he leaves us, we will have the memories and happy times as part of our own.

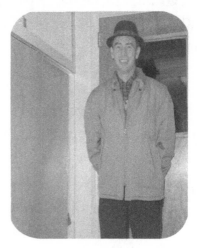

Hugh

I have sad news to relate concerning Hugh. He passed away at 3:52 a.m. on the 18th of June, 2016. He died peacefully at age 94. We are so glad we made the trip to visit him in January to tell him how much we loved him. We will miss him, but we will savor those happy memories.

Remembering Jum: by Minde Moore Connelly

What's For Dinner?

Vincent Price, the guy who starred in the Edgar Allan Poe movies, changed my life. Actually, Vincent did it through my father-in-law, Jum. In 1965, Vincent wrote a cookbook called "A Treasure of Great Recipes." A copy found its way into Jum's hands. It is a big heavy book and has gastronomic fame. Not a book for counting calories. Jum began making some of these recipes, which included Spaghetti Alla Bolognese. Can I tell you about this recipe? It has bacon, chicken livers, and cream. I grew up in a family of seven. Money was tight, and Mom did not go for fancy food. Dinner was meat and potatoes with corn or peas. When money was tight, we had canned tomatoes and milk or potato soup.

So when I married Jan, my Swedish/Italian/Irish husband, Jum, fixed us dinner. Yes, it was Spaghetti Alla Bolognese. I did not know about the complex combination of tomatoes, bacon, and cream. Or the careful cooking of spaghetti to a perfect al dente texture. The ladling of the spaghetti onto the plate by turning it slightly and neatly. Then, a fragrant and bountiful scoop of the sauce. I did not watch Jum prepare the sauce, and I regret having missed this experience.

I did watch him make his famous homemade bread. His bread was the type that exploded with flavor when toasted. There was an ongoing battle between Jum & Muz about how butter should be applied. Jum wanted the butter ice-cold, perhaps so it could melt slowly onto the golden crust, and Muz wanted the butter at room temperature. I do not believe either won.

Jum did not eat his food; he savored his food. It was a slow and deliberate process. Each bite was carefully measured. Chewing was accompanied by hums of contentment. And lastly, Jum would gesture with his thumb and index finger in a circle, bringing it to his mouth and quickly pull them away with an "ah-hh." I would wait for this ah-h. No one copied Jum's ah-hh because it was his and so genuine.

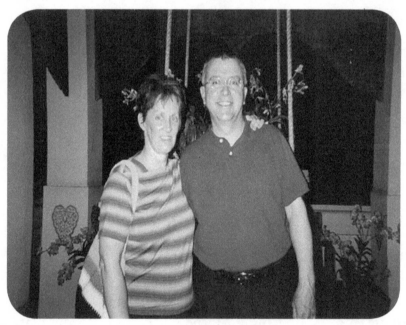

Minde and Jan

Information and Suggestions

More than 5 million Americans now have Alzheimer's disease. It is a fatal brain disease because it destroys the brain. It causes a slow decline in memory, thinking, and reasoning skills. It is the loss of mental and physicfunction that ultimately leads to death.

I am listing some of the warning signs I noticed in particular. You often forget recently learned information – names, appointments, telephone numbers. You forget simple tasks, such as cooking or getting dressed. You can't recall simple words and resort to descriptions, such as "that thing you drink out of" instead of a glass or repeating the same sentence or event over and over.

You notice changes in brain function that go beyond memory, such as confusion or agitation. Mood changes are an early symptom, which includes anxiety or depression. Personality changes, such as anger, unusual suspicions, or loss of motivation. The appearance of apathy, vagueness, not looking at you, eyes wandering.

I found some things that might help because the brain depends on strong circulation to stay healthy, eat right, choose good fats, and watch cholesterol. Maximize antioxidants from fruits and vegetables, vitamin C and E and B12– that neutralize the free radicals that kill brain cells and create the tangles. Drink alcohol in moderation. But, I think it is essential to help the damage to the brain's parts that control memory to control or reduce chronic stress. Stay active and do mental aerobics.

Probably the most important is to protect your head. Studies have confirmed that a concussion or a severe brain injury doubles the risk of Alzheimer's later in life. Some new drugs have been developed, either singly or in combination. There is no cure for Alzheimer's, but modern medications can slow its progression.

There is a difference between dementia and Alzheimers. In Alzheimer's, the motor skills also begin to deteriorate. Dementia can be caused by a combination of things, metabolism, infection, inflammation, or drug side effects. Addressing these improve cognitive function. Even people with Alzheimer's may see a marked improvement in skills.

Alzheimer's (AD) affects the whole body. It causes a slow decline in memory, thinking, and reasoning skills. Early diagnosis can help make decisions about future care. If Alzheimer's strikes, a doctor can review the symptoms and order tests such as an MRI (magnetic resonance imaging) to rule out other conditions such as a stroke or a tumor. A new test available is a PET (positron emission tomography) that can show damage even in the early stages. This test is costly – ranging from $700 to $1,500.

It's wise to have a neurological exam, especially if you have a family history of Alzheimer's. Studies have found that people who have the APOE epsilon4 allele (e4 gene) are at increased risk of developing Alzheimer's. However, exercise prevents brain shrinkage, so it's doubly important that people with the e4 gene exercise 2 or 3 times a week and, thus, will show dramatically less shrinkage.

1. Consistently low blood pressure can signal reduced blood flow to the brain, which raises the risk for older adults. Older brains are less able to compensate for the reduced blood flow and can lead to brain atrophy and dementia.

2. Chronic heartburn and the continuous use of antacids have a downside. Small studies have suggested that antacids cause a vitamin B-12 deficiency. They ruled out causes such as diabetes, thyroid disorders, smoking, and alcohol abuse. Vitamin B-12 is essential for brain function and your body's ability to make blood cells and DNA.

3. A recent study links hearing loss to dementia and Alzheimers. People with severe hearing loss are five times more likely to develop symptoms than those with normal hearing. But even mild hearing loss doubles the risk and triples among those with moderate hearing loss. As hearing worsens, the impaired person is more likely to become socially isolated, often leading to depression. This finding should prompt people to have their hearing checked. If necessary, fitted with appropriate hearing aids will keep them cognitively engaged and help preserve the brain and lessen the onset of Alzheimer's.

4. There is a growing body of evidence that inadequate sleep may be linked to Alzheimer's disease. Adequate sleep is crucial to overall health, and it's vitally essential for cognition, which relates to judgment, memory, and thinking. While scientists don't completely understand the connection, one theory examines the role of beta-amyloid. A toxic protein that builds up and forms plaques in the brain. Poor sleep may increase the risk for dementia, and dementia may interfere with the ability to sleep. Older individuals who wake frequently and those who get less than five hours of sleep demonstrated increased beta-amyloid. The precursor of Alzheimer's, says Dr. Robert Rosenberg, a board-certified sleep medicine physician.

5. A new research group is studying a possible connection between dementia and osteoporosis. Our physical strength and our mental aptitude are intertwined more than we realized. Researchers are uncovering some surprising links between two seemingly unrelated diseases. Having strong bones could help you maintain a sharp mind – and vice versa. Researchers in Germany evaluated data from 29,983 patients who had received an osteoporosis diagnosis over 20 years. They matched them with control agents, such as age, gender, index years, and several other diseases. The researchers found that 20.5% of the women with osteoporosis went on to receive a dementia diagnosis. Only 16.4% of the control group developed dementia, but this represents a 1.2-fold increase in risk. Now, this doesn't mean osteoporosis itself causes dementia. But, this increase gives us some strong hints about how we might treat both diseases. We can hone in on existing knowledge about these diseases.

6. New information about Alzheimer's research, a nasal spray that reduces Alzheimer's. Imagine a world where Alzheimer's is as rare as polio or smallpox. A breakthrough may be closer than you think. A recent study at Boston's Brigham and Women's Hospital, scientists gave subjects a nasal spray containing two drugs. Scientists expected the drugs to slow the growth of the brain plaques associated with Alzheimer's. What they didn't expect was that those memory-destroying plaques would simply disappear. During the 7-week study, amyloid plaques shrank by an astonishing 73%. Those kinds of results are unheard of, but when you look at the science behind the study, everything falls into place. This nasal spray activates a type

of brain cells known as microglia. Usually, these cells get rid of waste, remove dead cells, and clean up toxins. But they don't touch amyloid plaques. Until they get a dose of the treatment, overnight, these microglia turn into special forces snipers. And they lazer-target amyloid plaques and destroy them--while leaving other brain cells untouched. This study is extremely promising. And once this memory miracle gains FDA approval, Alzheimer's could soon become a thing of the past.

7. Two vitamins and minerals play critical roles in our bone and brain health. Vitamin K, our bones, need a form called K2 to make osteocalein. This protein hormone helps build bones and is also vital to brain health. Researchers have suggested that vitamin K deficiencies contribute to the pathogenesis of Alzheimer's. The vitamin seems to help protect neurons, particularly if you suffer from cardiovascular disease. Supplements may come with the "side effect" of strong bones. Patients with dementia are often at an increased risk of fractures in part because they're more likely to fall. The connection between vitamin K and dementia is not as well-established as between the vitamin and bone strength. Regardless, it's essential to maintain adequate levels of the vitamin for optimal health. Studies have confirmed that vitamin K directly affects the brain, whether or not a deficiency now causes AD. Vitamin K helps activate a gene called Gas6 and can protect neurons in the cerebral cortex from cell death due to amyloid plaques. This is a significant benefit. Vitamin K also helps the brain make sphingolipids. These lipids form part of the myelin sheath that coats the nerves as well as neurons cell membranes.

People should eat leafy greens and vegetables like asparagus and broccoli. A supplement should also contain vitamin D as well. Vitamin D also helps protect the central nervous system. It also helps limit the production of an enzyme that causes changes in neurons. And it promotes nerve growth. Studies have even found that vitamin D increases the expression of genes that slow AD progression. It also increases the number of amyloid-clearing macrophages in the brain. Clearly, vitamin D is vital in helping avoid both osteoporosis and dementia. Another ingredient is necessary; iron, this mineral, plays a key role in vitamin D metabolism. It is crucial to have a balanced diet. Vitamin D is a critical player in brain and bone health. Another study found that a severe vitamin D deficiency raises dementia risk by a whopping 125%. There's one final ingredient that helps effectively: iron. This mineral plays a crucial role in vitamin D metabolism. Taking a supplement is probably the safest way to have constant protection.

8. Advocates of stem cell research have raised public awareness and influenced decision-makers about vital research for Alzheimer's disease. The results have been promising. But the government should direct more money to research.

9. A breakthrough treatment suggests that symptoms of Alzheimer's might be reversed. A study published in the journal "Aging" presented an all-natural, multicomponent treatment program. The program is based on a new theory about why people get Alzheimer's, but this is new thinking and requires further study. It is showing promise in restoring memory.

The agenda, directed by Dale Bredesen, MD, is at the UCLA Alzheimers disease program. They have identified 36 factors affecting brain function. Addressing only one or two of these factors may not reverse memory loss. They have identified several key factors that may prevent, slow, stop, or potentially even turn back memory loss. They believe the more of these factors you incorporate into daily life, the more momentum there is to protect and restore memory. The theory, developed over two decades, of cellular and animal research at the Buck Institute for Research on Aging and UCLA.

An interesting study correlates a drug used to treat Diabetes might offer a treatment for Alzheimer's disease. The research will continue to be investigated and shows promise.

10 Early Warning Signs of Alzheimer's

1. Memory loss that disrupts daily life: Example: Forgetting recently learned information or asking the same question over and over.

2. Challenges in planning or solving problems: Example: Trouble keeping track of monthly bills.

3. Difficulty completing familiar tasks: Example: Having a hard time remembering the rules of a favorite card game.

4. Time or place confusion: Example: Forgetting how a destination was reached or where you are right now.

5. Trouble understanding visual images and spatial relationships: Example: Difficulty reading.

6. Problems with spoken or written word: Example: Repeating words.

7. Misplacing things and losing the ability to retrace steps: Example: Putting things in unusual places.

8. Decreased or poor judgment: Example: Paying less attention to personal grooming.

9. Withdrawal from work or social activities: Example: Avoiding social situations.

10. Changes in mood and personality: Example: Confusion, fearfulness, and anxiousness.

SOURCE: The Alzheimer's Association.

A final thought.

Remember: Occasional forgetfulness may be typical due to the lack of sleep or even dehydration that some of us experience from time to time. But if you consistently notice any of the symptoms listed above, be your best health advocate and make an appointment to see the doctor.

EPILOGUE

Following Jim's death, I spent a month in Wisconsin with Pat and his family. I flew with Sadie in a carrier. A soldier in uniform helped carry her on the way to the check-in. Arriving in Chicago to change planes, a man grabbed the carrier and said, "Come on, I'll help." A tale of how to win friends is to have a cute little dog.

The visit gave me time to rest and recover emotionally from the years of the struggle alongside Jim. I stayed in Washington State for a couple of years before moving to California in 2003. I spend my time gardening, reading, and watching favorite television programs. My daughter lives nearby, and my grandson Mike and his Children live close.

Sadie died of an auto-immune condition in January of 2015. She was sixteen years old, and I miss her. I have another dog, of course. They are the companions we need.

I live on the Calaveras River. It has steelhead and salmon, and the fish hang out in a deep hole just above some rapids. The area is abundant with wildlife, deer, mountain lions, raccoons, and almost anything you can name.

I lead a pleasant, restful life writing stories. I took a writing class, and my instructor suggested I put the stories into a book. The result was a collection of short stories about my family and growing up in Montana.

"Window to the Big Sky – Reflections from Montana," published in 2015.

Jan's wife Minde suggested the idea for this book. She thinks people will be interested in the Alzheimers story from the viewpoint of a caregiver. Perhaps it will help someone dealing with the disease. I believe this to be true.

When I started writing this book, I thought doing so would be cathartic, but it has had the opposite effect. It brought back all the hurt, anxiety, and loss that I experienced. Perhaps, those feelings will fade with time or at least be diminished over time. I hope so.

I do have a sense of optimism. I believe determination, strength, fortitude, and discovery will isolate, prevent, and maintain cognitive health. Great strides have already been achieved through research and studies. I have the belief that ultimately we will find a solution to the scourge of Alzheimer's.

Mary Ellen Connelly (Muz)